Surgical Strategies in Endourology for Stone Disease

Sanchia S. Goonewardene · Karen Ventii
Ali Gharib · Raymond J. Leveillee
David M. Albala

Surgical Strategies in Endourology for Stone Disease

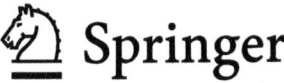 Springer

Sanchia S. Goonewardene
The Princess Alexandra Hospital
Department of Urology
Harlow, Essex
UK

Ali Gharib
The Princess Alexandra Hospital
Department of Urology
Harlow Essex
UK

David M. Albala
Urology
Associated Medical Professionals
Syracuse, NY
USA

Karen Ventii
Division of Urologic Surgery
Harvard University
Boston, MA
USA

Raymond J. Leveillee
Florida Atlantic University
Department of Surgery
Division of Urology
Bethesda Hospital
Baptist Health South Florida
Hollywood, FL
USA

ISBN 978-3-030-82145-6   ISBN 978-3-030-82143-2   (eBook)
https://doi.org/10.1007/978-3-030-82143-2

This Springer imprint is published by the registered company Springer Nature Switzerland AG
The registered company address is: Gewerbestrasse 11, 6330 Cham, Switzerland

Preface

Welcome to *Surgical Strategies in Endourology: Stone Disease* (SSIE). The concept of this book first came to me as a young trainee whilst learning stone surgery. Endourology is a critical area of urology, often with very sick patients. In endourological treatments, there are clearly a myriad of choices to be made, both relating to equipment and relating to key steps within each procedure. What are the right choices and why do experienced endourologists do what they do?

Endourology is a core component of urological practice. Within this book, we have pulled together interesting cases that enable you to further develop your decision-making skills. This subspeciality in urology is often unpredictable and has many pitfalls. The most important lesson to take away from this is to understand that many options exist in treating stones and making the correct choices matters. Prevention is far better than a cure.

We hope you will find this book both informative and enjoyable.

Harlow, UK   Sanchia S. Goonewardene
Cambridge, MA   Karen Ventii
Harlow, UK   Ali Gharib
Boynton Beach, FL   Raymond J. Leveillee
Syracuse, NY   David M. Albala

Acknowledgements

For my family and friends, and work family, for always supporting me in what I do.

For all the superheroes in my life, who have supported me.

For my team at Springer Nature, for always giving myself and my team a chance to get published.

For the amazing Associate Prof Khalid Shehzad, all credit for the beautifully drawn illustrations goes to him.

For Karen Ventii, I could not wish for a more perfect copy editor.

For Ali Gharib, the best Clinical Lead and Head of Department.

For Raymond J Leveillee, thank you for the time and effort, all credit for the amazing photos goes to him.

For my mentor, coach, Editor-in-Chief, Prof David Albala, I could not have achieved all of this without you.

Abbreviations

A+E	Accident and Emergency
AF	Atrial Fibrillation
AKI	Acute Kidney Injury
B-TURP	Bipolar TURP
BAUS	British Association of Urological Surgeons
BCG	Bacille Calmette-Guerin
BMI	Body Mass Index
BPH	Benign Prostatic Hyperplasia
CA	Cancer
CAOX	Calcium Oxalate
CT	Computer Tomography
CT KUB	CT Kidneys Ureter Bladder
CVA	Cerebrovascular Accident
DRE	Digital Rectal Exam
DVT	Deep Venous Thrombosis
DXT	Radiotherapy
EAU	European Association of Urology
ESWL	Extracorporeal Shockwave Lithotripsy
EUA	Examination under Anaesthesia
FURS	Flexible Ureterorenoscopy
HDU	High Dependency Unit
HOLEP	Holmium Laser Enucleation of the Prostate
INR	Internal Normalised Ratio
IPSS	International Prostate Symptom Score
ITU	Intensive Care Unit
IVP	Intravenous Pyelogram
IVU	Intravenous Urogram
LNU	Laparoscopic Nephroureterectomy
LOS	Length of Stay
LUTS	Lower Urinary Tract Symptoms
NSAIDs	Nonsteroidal Anti-Inflammatory Drugs
MI	Myocardial Infarction
MET	Medical Expulsive Therapy
MMC	Mitomycin C

MRI	Magnetic Resonance Imaging
NICE	National Institute for Clinical Excellence
ONU	Open Nephroureterectomy
PAE	Prostate Artery Embolisation
PCNL/PNL	Percutaneous Nephrolithotomy
PE	Pulmonary Embolism
PTH	Parathyroid Hormone
PUJ/PUJO	Pelviureteric Junction Obstruction
PVR	Post-Void Residual
SR	Systematic Review
SWL	Shock Wave Lithotripsy
TCC	Transitional Cell Carcinoma
TFTS	Thyroid Function Tests
TURBT	Transurethral Resection of Bladder Tumour
TURP	Transurethral Resection of the Prostate
TWOC	Trial without Catheter
UDS	Urodynamics
UO	Ureteric Orifice
URS	Ureteroscopy
US	Ultrasound Scan
UTI	Urinary Tract Infection
UUT-TCC	Upper Urinary Tract Transitional Cell Carcinoma
VUJ	Vesicoureteric Junction
XRAY KUB	Kidneys Ureter Bladder

Contents

About the Authors

Sanchia S. Goonewardene, MBChB BMedSc PGCGC Dip.SSC MRCS qualified from Birmingham Medical School with Honours in Clinical Science and a BMedSc Degree in Medical Genetics and Molecular Medicine. She has a specific interest in academia during her spare time, with over 727 publications to her credit with 2 papers as the number 1 most cited in fields (Biomedical Library), and has significantly contributed to the Urological Academic World—she has since added a section to the European Association of Urology Congress on Prostate Cancer Survivorship and Supportive Care and has been an associate member of an EAU guidelines panel on Chronic Pelvic Pain (2015–2021). She has been the UK lead in an EAU-led study on salvage prostatectomy. She has also contributed to the BURST IDENTIFY study as a collaborator. Her background with research entails an MPhil, the work from which went on to be drawn up as a document for PCUK then, endorsed by NICE. She gained funding from the Wellcome Trust for her research elective. She is also an alumnus of the Urology Foundation, who sponsored a trip to USANZ trainee week. She also has 6 books published—Core Surgical Procedures for Urology Trainees, Prostate Cancer Survivorship, Basic Urological Management, Management of Non-Muscle Invasive Bladder Cancer, Salvage Therapy in Prostate Cancer, and Management of Muscle Invasive Bladder Cancer. She has supervised her first thesis with King's College London and Guys Hospital (BMedSci Degree; gained first class and students' thesis score 95%). She is an Associate Editor for the Journal of Robotic Surgery and is responsible as Urology Section Editor. She is an editorial board member of the World Journal of Urology and was invited to be Guest Editor for a Special Issue on Salvage Therapy in Prostate Cancer. She is also a review board member for BMJ case reports. Additionally, she is on the International Continence Society Panel on Pelvic Floor Dysfunction and Good Urodynamic Practice Panel, is an ICS abstract reviewer, and has been an EPoster Chair at ICS. More recently, she has been an ICS Ambassador and is an ICS Mentor. She has also chaired semi-live surgery at ERUS and presented her work as part of the Young Academic Urology Section at ERUS. In her spare time, she enjoys fundraising for Rotary International and is Secretary and Vice President (President Elect 2022–2023) for the Rotary Club of Hampstead. Most recently, she is mentoring a PhD student, with Roteract.

Karen H. Ventii, BSc, MSc, PhD is a Harvard-trained specialist in healthcare communications, with over 10 years of experience in oncology and urology. As a Visiting Fellow at Harvard University, she conducted independent research on evolving trends in continuing medical education, with the aim of diminishing the gap between evidence and practice. Her research was conducted in collaboration with Dr. Aria F. Olumi (Janet and William DeWolf Professor of Surgery/Urology at Harvard Medical School, Chief of Urologic Surgery at Beth Israel Deaconess Medical Center, and Chair of Research for the American Urological Association).

Throughout her career, Dr. Ventii has demonstrated excellence on numerous medical education initiatives in the academic and pharmaceutical sectors, including the NIH Broadening Experience in Scientific Training (BEST) initiative to enhance training opportunities for early career scientists and prepare them for career options in the dynamic biomedical workforce landscape. Dr. Ventii has also authored many oncology- and urology-focused publications including a review article on "Biomarkers in Prostate Cancer" which was selected as one of the top oncology reviews of 2014.

Dr. Ventii has worked with several global healthcare companies focused on oncology and has been responsible for content development, content editing, publications, and supporting strategic planning on several accounts.

Dr. Ventii holds a doctorate in biochemistry from Emory University in Atlanta, GA, and a Bachelor of Science as well as a Master of Science in Biology from Duquesne University in Pittsburgh, PA. Upon completing her doctorate, she continued her research efforts at the Winship Cancer Institute investigating the biochemical properties of the breast cancer-associated protein-1 (BAP1) tumour suppressor protein. Her research has been published in peer-reviewed journals such as *Cancer Research*, *Biochemistry*, and *Oncology* and she has presented her work in oral and poster formats at national conferences.

Ali Gharib, MBBS, MD completed his urology training and residency at Kaunas Medical University Hospital, Lithuania, as a qualified urologist in the EU performing radical prostatectomy, cystoprostatectomies, and nephrectomies. On GMC'S specialist register since 2011, he was appointed as a urologist at Milton Keynes University Hospital. In 2018, as a Consultant at King's College University Hospitals at Princess Royal University Hospital site. His clinical interests focused mainly on urinary stones disease and prostate cancer in addition to other interests including bladder cancer as well as andrology.

After being a Urology Consultant at King's College University Hospitals, Gharib was appointed as Consultant Urologist at Princess Alexandra Hospital NHS Trust. He is currently the Clinical Lead for Urology Department at Princess Alexandra Hospital NHS Trust.

Raymond J. Leveillee, MD, FRCS completed his residency in Urology at Brown University before commencing with an Endourology/Laparoscopy fellowship from the renowned Department of Urology at the University of Minnesota in 1995. He rose to the rank of a tenured professor at the University of Miami over a 20-year period. He held appointments in the Departments of Urology, Radiology, and Biomedical Engineering with mentorship for fellows in the Endourology Society. He is considered a world leader in robotics, kidney and prostate cancer, obstructive uropathies, endourology, and complex stone disease. A pioneer and outward thinker for his entire career, Dr. Leveillee has been afforded international acclaim being given the distinction of induction into the Thai Urological Society under the Royal Patronage and receiving a medical degree "Ad Eundem" from the Royal College of Surgeons in Glasgow (Scotland). Politically motivated and savvy, he was in the inaugural class of the American Urological Association (AUA) Leadership program, has served on numerous AUA committees including Practice Guidelines, and is Past President of both the Florida Urological Society and Southeastern Section of AUA (SESAUA). He presently serves on AUA Kidney and Adrenal Health Committee and is the Alternate Representative to the AUA Board of Directors. Dr. Leveillee currently is the Director of the BETHESDA CENTER FOR ADVANCED ROBOTICS AND UROLOGIC CARE (a post he has held since August 2015) and is an affiliate Professor of Surgery/Urology at the Charles C. Schmidt College of Medicine at Florida Atlantic University.

David M. Albala, MD graduated with a geology degree from Lafayette College in Easton, Pennsylvania. He completed his medical school training at Michigan State University and went on to complete his surgical residency at the Dartmouth-Hitchcock Medical Centre. Following this, Dr. Albala was an endourology fellow at Washington University Medical Centre under the direction of Ralph V. Clayman. He practised at Loyola University Medical Centre in Chicago and rose from the ranks of Instructor to full Professor in Urology and Radiology in 8 years. After 10 years, he became a tenured Professor at Duke University Medical Centre in North Carolina. At Duke, he was Co-Director of the Endourology fellowship and Director for the Centre of Minimally Invasive and Robotic Urological Surgery. He has over 180 publications in peer-reviewed journals and has authored six books in endourology and general urology. He is the Editor-in-Chief of the Journal of Robotic Surgery. He serves on the editorial board for Medical Reviews in Urology, Current Opinions in Urology, and Urology Index and Reviews. He serves as a reviewer for eight surgical journals. Presently, he is Chief of Urology at Crouse Hospital in Syracuse, New York, and a physician at Associated Medical Professionals (a group of 33 urologists). He is considered a national and international authority in laparoscopic and robotic urological surgery and has been an active teacher in this area for over 20 years. His research and clinical interests have focused on robotic urological surgery. In addition, other clinical interests include minimally invasive treatment of benign prostatic hypertrophy (BPH), stone disease, and the use of fibrin sealants in surgery. He has been a Visiting Professor at numerous institutions across the USA as well as overseas in countries such as India, China, England, Iceland, Germany, France, Japan, Brazil, Australia, and Singapore. In addition, he has done operative demonstrations in over 32 countries and 23 states. He has trained 16 fellows in endourology and advanced robotic surgery. In addition, Dr. Albala is a past White House Fellow who acted as a special assistant to Federico Pena, Secretary of Transportation, on classified and unclassified public health-related issues.

Types of Stone Treatment

1

1.1   Management Options for Stones

Management options
- Shock wave lithotripsy- shockwaves delivered to a single stone in a non obstructed patient, with no acute kidney injury and not septic.
- Stones must be 10 mm or less and patients must not be obstructed.
- Percutaneous nephrostolithotomy- usually done for large stone burdens in the kidney, staghorn stones, or 2-3 cm renal stones.
- Ureteroscopy- can be used for stones up to 1.5 mm.
- Conservative management- usually done for small (<5mm) symptomatic renal stones or stones in a non-obstructive position. (Tables 1.1 and 1.2)

NICE and EAU Guidelines on Conservative management
- Conservative management can be used if the stone is less than 5 mm or if the stone is larger than 5 mm and the person (or their family or care givers) agrees (NICE, Guidelines, 2019).
- Conservative observational management of renal stones is possible, although the availability of minimally invasive treatment often leads to active treatment (Turk, 2016, EAU Guidelines on Urolithiasis).
- Ureteral stones <6mm can pass spontaneously in well-controlled patients (TURK,2016)
- Acute renal colic due to ureteral stone obstruction is an emergency that requires immediate pain management.
- Mechanical Expulsion Therapy (MET), usually with α-receptor antagonists, facilitates stone passage and reduces the need for analgesia

Endoscopic
- Began in late 1979
- Now the main stay of practice
- Technological advances and changing treatment patterns have had an impact on current treatment (Turk, 2016b).
- Active treatment of urolithiasis is currently a minimally invasive intervention, with a preference for endourologic techniques (Turk, 2 016b).
- For active removal of stones from the kidney or ureter, technological advances have made it possible to use less invasive surgical techniques.

Shock Wave Lithotripsy Era
- First lithotripters available 1984-1985
- Introduced in 1980s
  - Christian Chaussy, MD and Egbert Schmiedt,
  - The Dornier HM3 lithotripter- an Electrohydraulic lithotripter
- Release of energy from a capacitor (spark gap) in μsecs
- Now treatment choice for majority of small non-obstructive stones
- As per NICE guidance, patients are not stented pre ESWL, only consider if they are children or young adults with staghorn stones (NICE Guidance, 2019).

Conservative treatment
- Stones < 2mm
  - 8.2 days on average to pass
- Stones 2 to 4mm
  - 12.2 days on average to pass
- Stones 4 to 6mm
  - 22 days on average to pass
  - (Miller & Kane, 1999)

© The Author(s), under exclusive license to Springer Nature Switzerland AG 2021
S. S. Goonewardene et al., *Surgical Strategies in Endourology for Stone Disease*, https://doi.org/10.1007/978-3-030-82143-2_1

Table 1.1 Demonstrating changing treatment

Type of treatment	1980s	1990s	2000s
Shock wave lithotripsy	95%	85%	75%
Endoscopic Procedure	5%	15%	25%
Open stone Surgery	<1%	<1%	<1%

Miller and Kane (1999)

Table 1.2 Average days to stone passage

Size of stone	Average days to stone passage
2 mm	7 days
3 mm	12 days
4 mm	23 days

Miller and Kane (1999)

1.2   NICE Guidelines on Stones

NICE Guidelines 2019 on stones

- Diagnostics in stone disease
- Offer urgent (within 24 hours of presentation) low-dose non-contrast CT to adults with suspected renal colic. If a woman is pregnant, offer an ultrasound instead of CT.

Offer urgent ultrasound (within 24 hours) as first-line imaging for children and young people with suspected renal colic.
If there is still uncertainty about the diagnosis of renal colic after ultrasound for children and young people, consider low-dose non-contrast CT.

1.3   Outcomes from Stone Management

An increase in minimally invasive techniques has led to the decrease in open surgery (Srisubat, 2014). Extracorporeal shock wave lithotripsy (ESWL) has been introduced as an alternative approach which disintegrates stones in the kidney and upper urinary tract through the use of shock waves (Srisubat, 2014). Nevertheless, as there are limitations with the success rate in ESWL, other minimally invasive modalities for kidney stones such as percutaneous nephrolithotomy (PCNL) and retrograde intrarenal surgery (RIRS) are also widely applied (Srisubat, 2014).

The success of treatment at three months was significantly greater in the PCNL compared to the ESWL group in patients with large stone burden (3 studies, 201 participants: RR 0.46, 95% CI 0.35 to 0.62) (Srisubat, 2014). Re-treatment (1 study, 122 participants: RR 1.81, 95% CI 0.66 to 4.99) and using auxiliary procedures (2 studies, 184 a: RR 9.06, 95% CI 1.20 to 68.64) was significantly increased with ESWL group compared to PCNL (Srisubat, 2014).

Duration of treatment (MD -36.00 min, 95% CI -54.10 to -17.90) and hospital stay (1 study, 49 participants: MD -3.30 days, 95% CI -5.45 to -1.15) were significantly shorter in the ESWL group (Srisubat, 2014). Overall more complications were reported with PCNL, however we were unable to meta-analyse the included studies due to the differing outcomes reported and the timing of the outcome measurements (Srisubat, 2014). One study compared ESWL versus RIRS for lower pole kidney stones. The success of treatment was not significantly different at the end of the third month (58 participants: RR 0.91, 95% CI 0.64 to 1.30) (Srisubat, 2014).

References

Guidelines NICE. Renal and ureteric stones. BJUI. 2019;123(2):220–32.

Türk C, Petřík A, Sarica K, Seitz C, Skolarikos A, Straub M, Knoll T. EAU Guidelines on diagnosis and conservative Management of Urolithiasis. Eur Urol. 2016 Mar;69(3):468–74.

Türk C, Petřík A, Sarica K, Seitz C, Skolarikos A, Straub M, Knoll T. EAU Guidelines on interventional treatment for urolithiasis. Eur Urol. 2016b Mar;69(3):475–82.

Miller OF. Kane CJ time to stone passage for observed ureteral calculi: a guide for patient education. J Urol. 1999 Sep;162(3 Pt 1):688–9.

Srisubat A, Potisat S, Lojanapiwat B, Setthawong V, Laopaiboon M. Extracorporeal Shock Wave Lithotripsy (ESWL) Versus Percutaneous Nephrolithotomy (PCNL) or Retrograde Intrarenal Surgery (RIRS) for Kidney Stones. Cochrane Database Syst Rev. 2014;11:CD007044.

Percutaneous Nephrolithotomy (PCNL)

2

2.1   Role and Indication of PCNL

Role of PCNL

- Though PCNL comes with higher morbidity, its efficacy is greater than other minimally invasive modalities for large stone burdens.
- Potential complications such as bleeding and hydrothorax can occur. (Knoll, 2017)
- Uses of PCNL:
- <u>Large Stone Size</u>- Staghorn calculi
- <u>Stone Location</u>- Stones in calyceal diverticulum, Horseshoe kidney, Lower pole calculi >1cm.
- <u>Hard Stone Composition</u>- Cystine, CaOx Monohydrate.

Indication

- Stone Volume
- Stones >3cm diameter, stones 2-3cm in diameter (where preferred to ESWL with JJ stenting or URS), staghorn stones, lower pole stones >1cm
- Obesity precluding SWL, failed other modalities
- Distal obstruction preventing passage of stone fragments.
- Hard stones- Cystine composition
- Modern-day PCNL allows personalized stone management tailored to individual patient and surgeon factors. (Ghani, 2016)

Special considerations

- PCNL is associated with higher stone-free rates at the expense of higher complication rates, blood loss, and admission times (De, 2015).
- There is a risk of bleeding which may require transfusion, renal embolisation or rarely nephrectomy.
- It is very often conducted in the prone position
- Pulmonary complications can occur (pneumothorax, haemothorax, urinothorax) requiring chest drain
- It is technology dependent-Fluoroscopy and ultrasound experience helpful
- Bowel perforation-small risk in female, thin patients

Imaging modalities

- Image guidance is a critical factor for the performance of urologic interventions. (Kalogeropoulou, 2009)
- Fluoroscopy
- Commenest- good overview of calyceal anatomy
- Ultrasonography- realtime access, sector view
- CT guided- very precise anatomy and puncture

2.2　Contraindications to PCNL

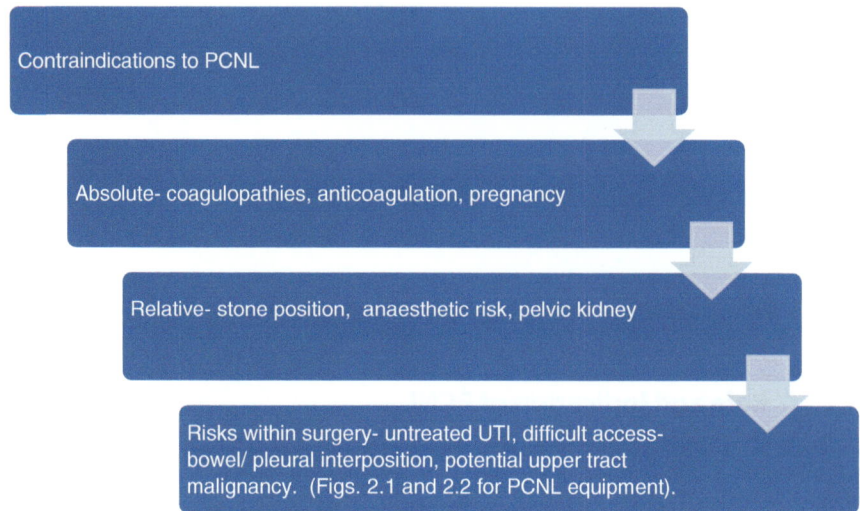

Contraindications to PCNL

Absolute- coagulopathies, anticoagulation, pregnancy

Relative- stone position, anaesthetic risk, pelvic kidney

Risks within surgery- untreated UTI, difficult access-bowel/ pleural interposition, potential upper tract malignancy. (Figs. 2.1 and 2.2 for PCNL equipment).

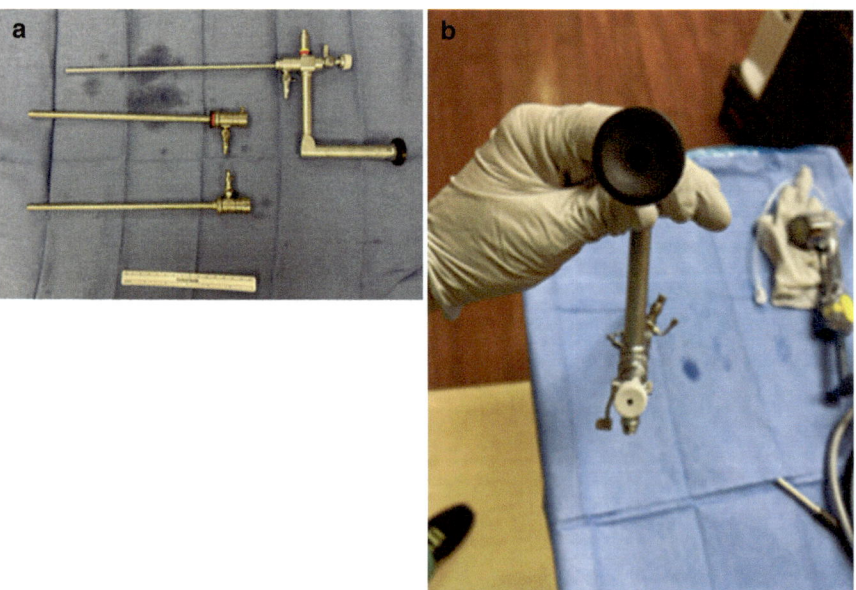

Fig. 2.1 (**a** and **b**) The nephroscope with 24 fr and 26 fr sheaths

Fig. 2.2 Fluroscopy
during PCNL

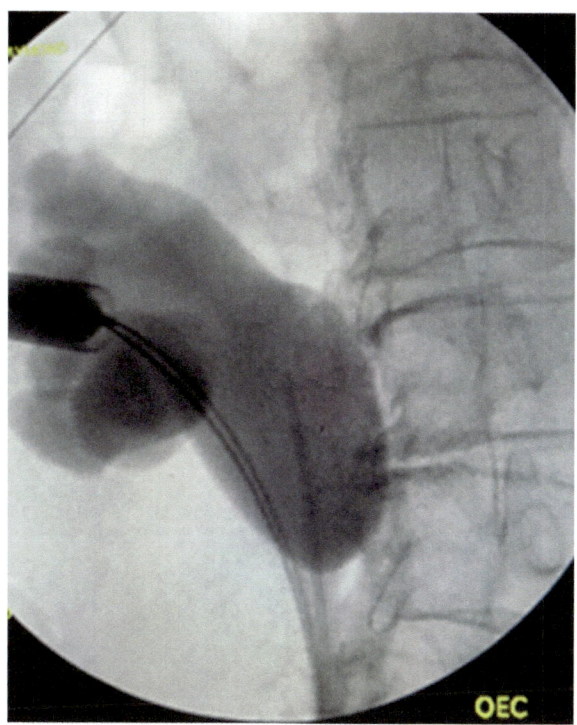

2.3   PCNL complications (BAUS, 2019)

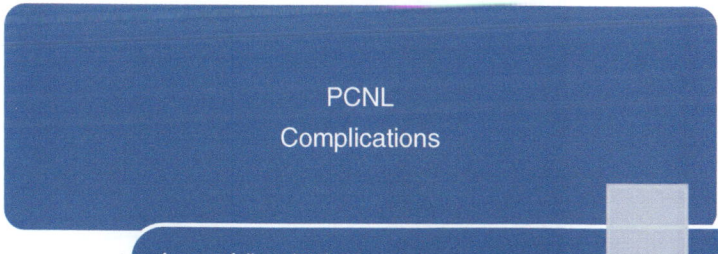

PCNL
Complications

- Access failure (5%)
- Bleeding requiring transfusion (11%), requiring embolisation (1%)
- Perforation of adjacent organs (bowel <1%, pneumothorax 0.5%)
- Pleural effusion (10%)
- Residual stones (>10%)
- Infection (sepsis 0.25-1.5%)
- Mortality (0.3%)
- Nephrectomy (<1%) (Figs. 2.3, 2.4 and 2.5).

Complications	Trans-fusion	Embolisation	Urinoma	Fever	Sepsis	Thoracic complication	Organ injury	Death	LE
(Range)	(0-20%)	(0-1.5%)	(0-1%)	(0-32.1%)	(0.3-1.1%)	(0-11.6%)	(0-1.7%)	(0-0.3%)	1a
N = 11,929	7%	0.4%	0.2%	10.8%	0.5%	1.5%	0.4%	0.05%	

Fig. 2.3 Complications of PCNL, EAU Guidelines on Urolithiasis, 2019

Fig. 2.4 PCNL can be used in complex renal calculi- preop KUB

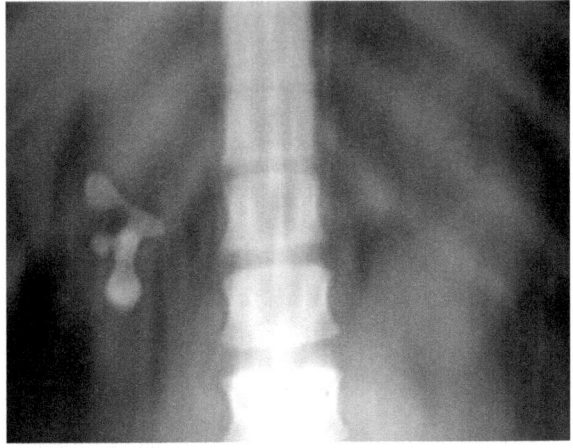

Fig. 2.5 Pre op IVU

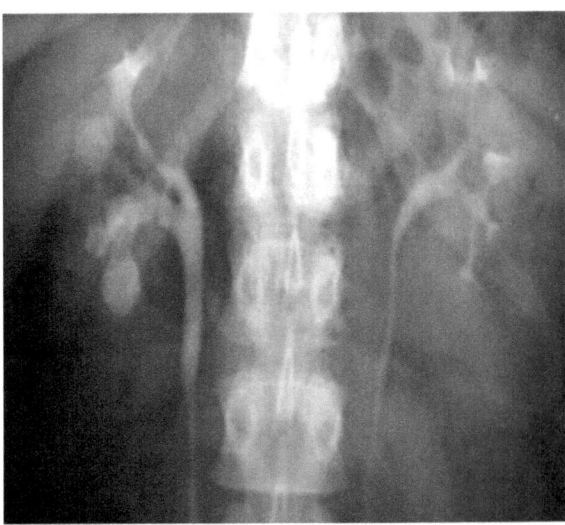

2.4 Modern Role of PCNL in Stone Surgery

Since the first successful stone extraction through a nephrostomy in 1976, percutaneous nephrolithotomy (PCNL) has become the preferred procedure especially for treatment of large, complex and staghorn calculi (Lucarelli, 2013). Most PCNL are performed with the patient in a prone position. More recently, particular interest has been taken on supine PCNL due to fewer anestesiological risks and the possibility of simultaneous anterograde and retrograde access to the whole urinary tract (Lucarelli, 2013).

Although many retrospective studies have been published, only two prospective trials comparing the two positions are reported in the literature (Lucarelli, 2013). The best access to PCNL is still a controversial issue. The overall experience reported in the literature indicates that each approach is equally feasible and safe and guided by physician experience (Lucarelli, 2013).

References

De S, Autorino R, Kim FJ, Zargar H, Laydner H, Balsamo R, Torricelli FC, Di Palma C, Molina WR, Monga M, De Sio M. Percutaneous nephrolithotomy versus retrograde intrarenal surgery: a systematic review and meta-analysis. Eur Urol. 2015 Jan;67(1):125–37.

Ghani KR, Andonian S, Bultitude M, Desai M, Giusti G, Okhunov Z, Preminger GM, de la Rosette J. Percutaneous Nephrolithotomy: update, trends, and future directions. Eur Urol. 2016 Aug;70(2):382–96.

Kalogeropoulou C, Kallidonis P, Liatsikos EN. Imaging in percutaneous nephrolithotomy. J Endourol. 2009 Oct;23(10):1571–7.

Knoll T, Daels F, Desai J, Hoznek A, Knudsen B, Montanari E, Scoffone C, Skolarikos A, Tozawa K. Percutaneous nephrolithotomy: technique. World J Urol. 2017 Sep;35(9):1361–8.

Lucarelli G, Breda A. Prone and Supine Percutaneous Nephrolithotomy. Minerva Urol Nefrol. 2013;65(2):93–9.

Access for PCNL: Which Calyx and How to Puncture

3.1 Types of PCNL Access, Calyceal Punctures, Equipment

Types of access
- Fluoroscopic guidance-xray guided vs. Ultrasound guidance- using ultrasound
- Retrograde access catheter or balloon catheter- to obstruct ureter
- Supracostal punctures (for upper pole access) vs subcostal (for lower pole access)
- Calyceal access only
- Supine vs. prone position
- (Kalogeropoulou, 2009)

Which calyx
- Traditionally, a lower pole access was routinely performed for less complication.
- Upper calyces are also preferred for access in a given condition with large and complex calculi (Zeng, 2015).
- Influence by calyx and technique selected, and the ribs, also shortest skin to calyx distance.

Puncture technique
- Bull eye technique (A. Smith)- perc onto stone
- 2 planes adjustment technique (Lingeman, 2005) - Cross reference two planes, to get access. (Figs. 3.1, 3.2 and 3.3).

Equipment required
- Rigid nephroscope
- Flexible nephroscope
- Ultrasonic device
- Pneumatic device
- Flexible ureteroscope

© The Author(s), under exclusive license to Springer Nature Switzerland AG 2021
S. S. Goonewardene et al., *Surgical Strategies in Endourology for Stone Disease*,
https://doi.org/10.1007/978-3-030-82143-2_3

Fig. 3.1 The PCNL
access set

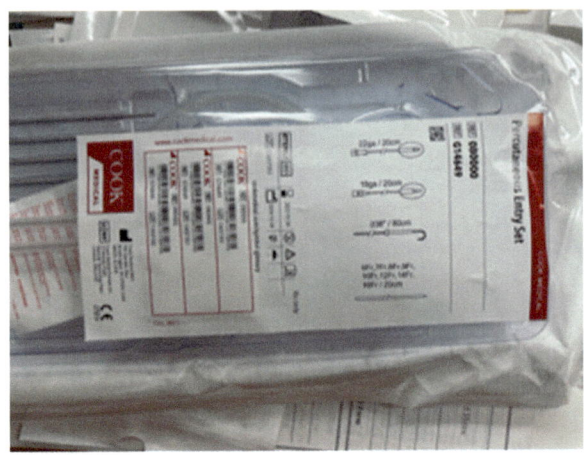

Fig. 3.2 PCNL Dilators-
for dilation of tract

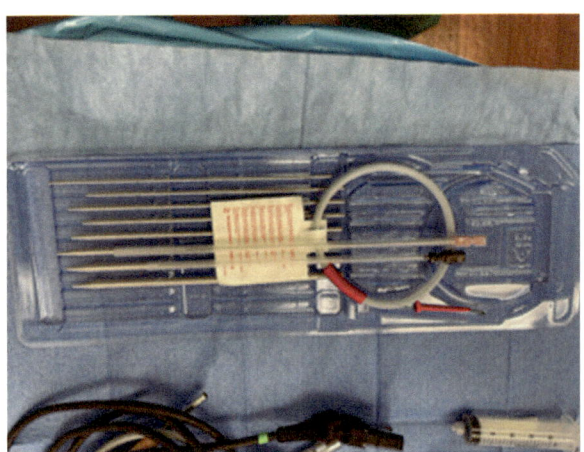

Fig. 3.3 Needle setup for puncture down onto a stone

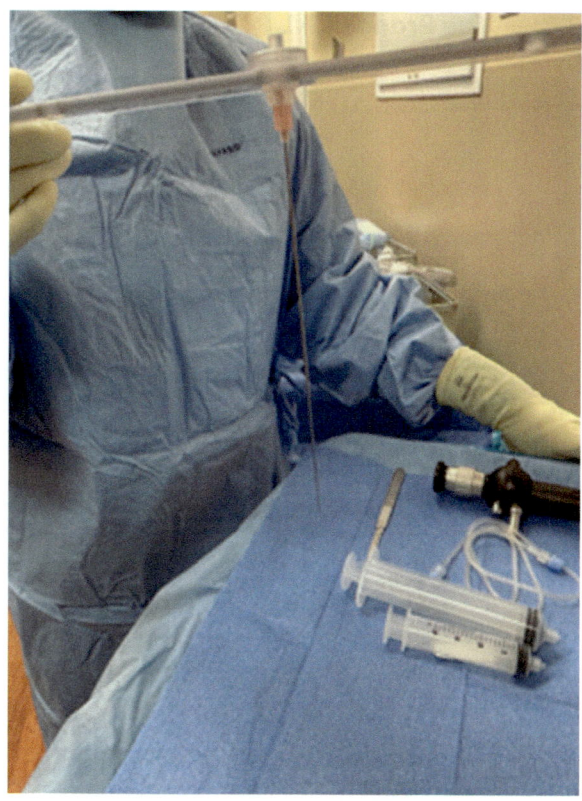

3.2   Peri-Operative Assessment for PCNL

Prior to PCNL

Assess CT
For stone position, location, position of calyces- look for shortest skin to stone distance
Also assess position of bowel, liver/spleen and pleura

Check Medical history- look for fitness for GA and anticoagulants
Check bloods- assess for coagulopathies beforehand
Urine culture- make sure patient does not have untreated UTI

Rivera (2016)

3.3　The Prone PCNL Puncture

Prone puncture

- Rigid cystoscopy - conduct a retrograde pyelogram to highlight the collecting system
- Once the calyx for access has been identified, rotate the C arm in 20-30 degrees in axial plane
- Posterior calyx usually more opaque on retrograde

- Under image guidance, place the needle onto the stone- the calyx has been entered if the needle moves with respiration
- Remove the stylet to visualise urine/blue dye
- Wire inserted into pelvis/down ureter into bladder with double lumen catheter for second working wire
- Safety wire secured through and through
- Skin incision and tract dilation to 24-30F for standard PCNL using either balloon, serial metal or amplatz dilators
- Advantages of balloon dilation of tract: Blood loss, Transfusion rates, LOS, and Recovery time. (Figs. 3.4 and 3.5).

Fig. 3.4 The Position for
Prone PCNL

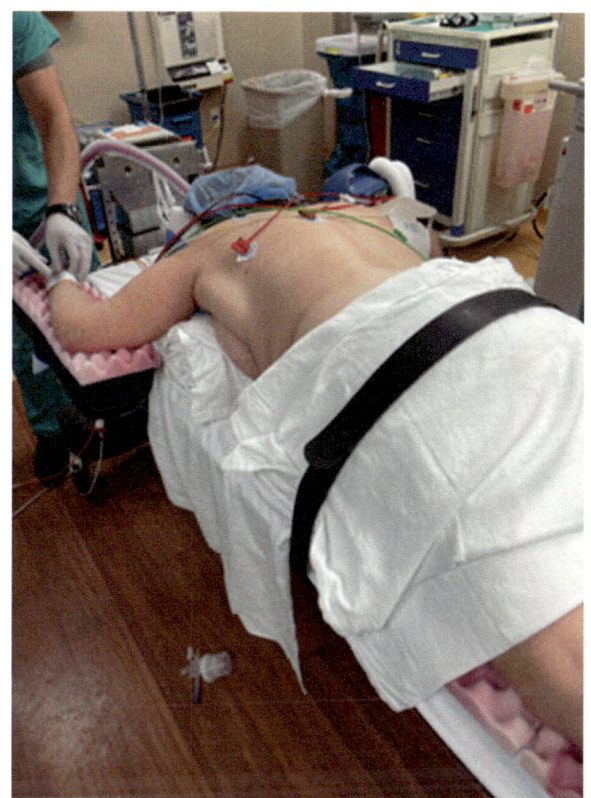

Fig. 3.5 The C- Arm-used
in stone surgery to
visualise stones

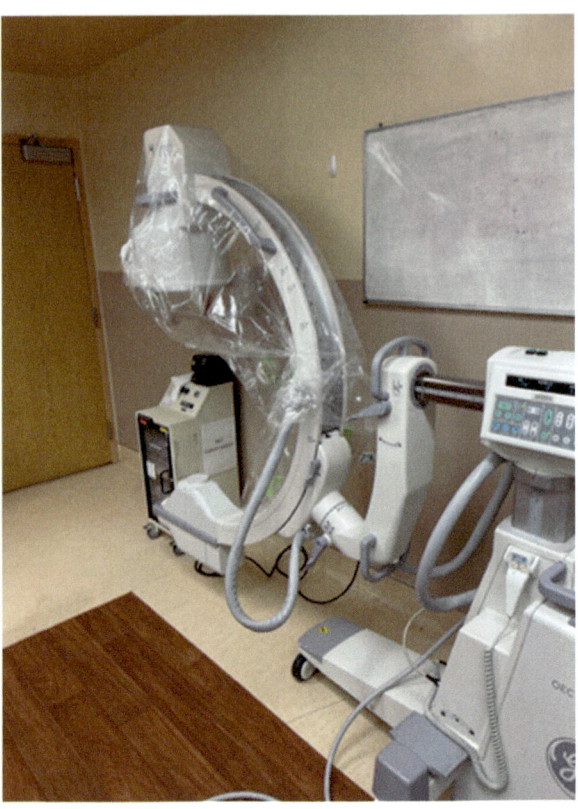

3.4 Supine vs. Prone PCNL: Which Is Better?

Prone position

- Most common procedure
- Medially placed puncture
- Access posterior calyx more easily
- Patel, 2017

Disadvantages of prone procedure

- Need to turn patient in procedure
- Airway management - often difficult to access during procedure, should there be airway issues
- Venous return- poor in the prone positions
- Patel, 2017

Supine Position

- Newer procedure
- Anaesthetics- the airway is well protected
- Can do endoscopic combined procedure
- Low pressure in collecting system- less risk of perforating a calyx
- Patel, 2017

Disadvantages of Supine procedure

- Greater learning curve, especially if used to prone
- Higher risk of visceral injury compared to prone
- Smaller operative field
- Patel, 2017 (Figs. 3.6, 3.7, 3.8, 3.9 and 3.10 for PCN L access)

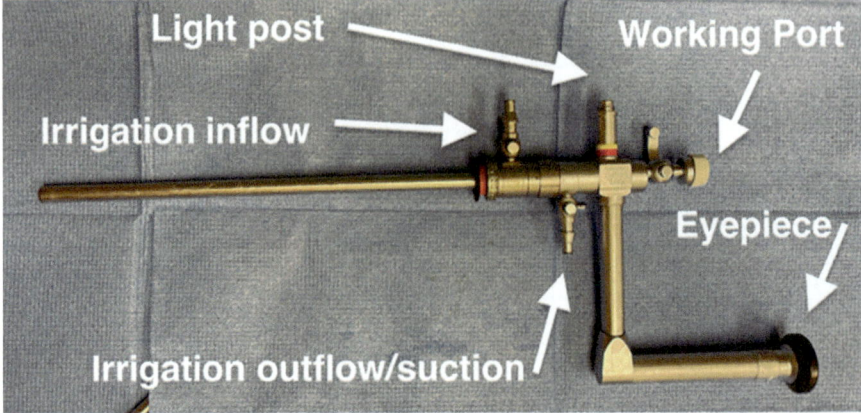

Fig. 3.6 The Nephroscope

Fig. 3.7 Staghorn on
Xray- operated on with
Nephroscope

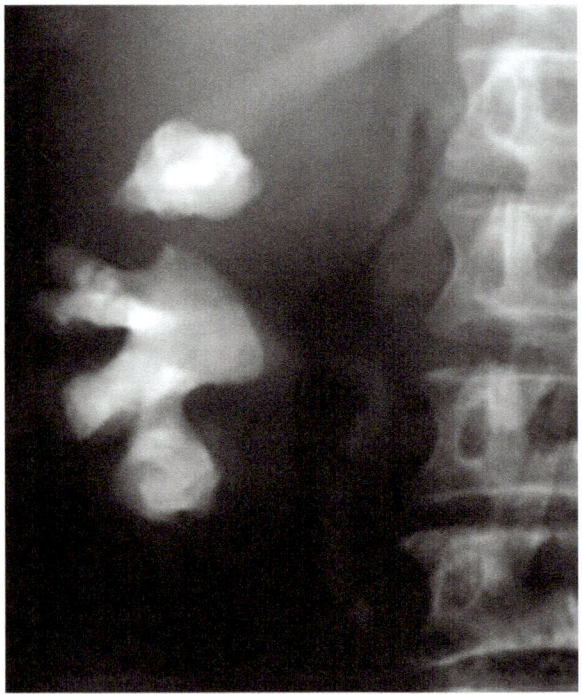

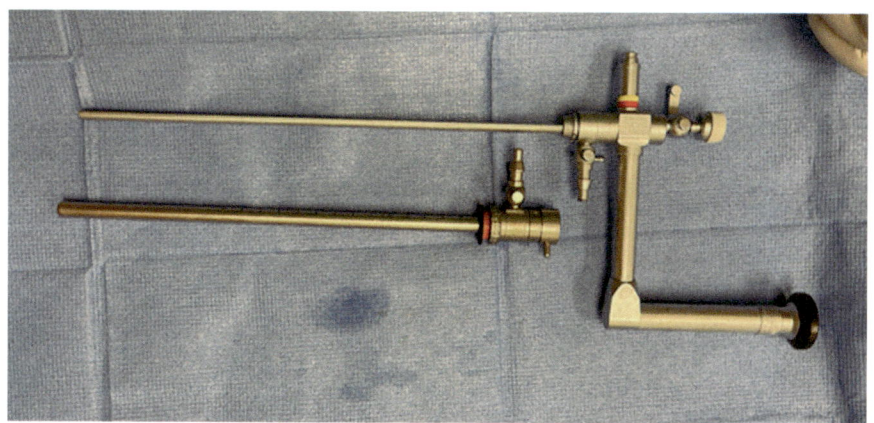

Fig. 3.8 Rigid Nephroscope Lens and Sheath

Fig. 3.9 Staghorn stone on KUB

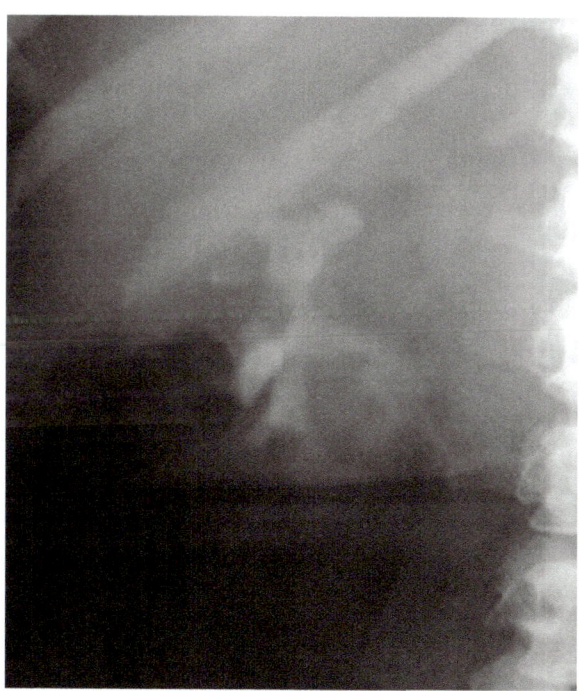

Fig. 3.10 Retrograde
renal access. To minimize
pleural morbidity, tubeless
upper-pole access should
be considered if the kidney
is judged to be stone free at
the conclusion of PCNL

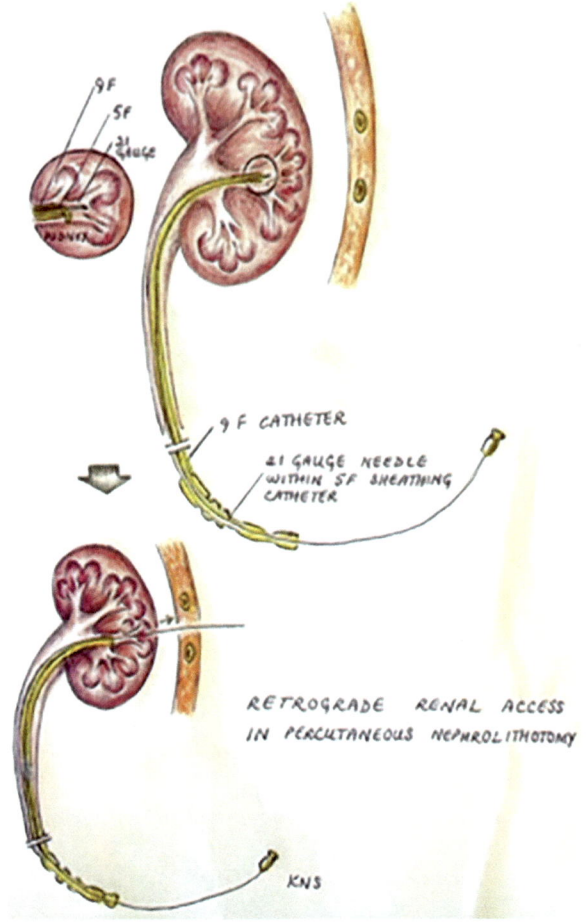

3.5   Types of Lithotripsy in PCNL

Options for stone removal

- Intracorporeal lithotripsy-pneumatic, ultrasonic, combination
- Holmium laser
- Fragmentation and forceps removal

Ultrasonic lithotripsy

- First described to fragment renal calculi in 1979
- Hollow probe (2.5 ~ 4 F)
    Has advantage of "vacuum" capabilities
- High frequency (> 20 kHz) mechanical vibration generated by piezoelectric transducers
- "Drilling and grinding" of the target stone

Pneumatic lithotripsy

- Pneumatically driven piston fragments stones by direct contact
- Major advantages: Improved efficacy
                       Multiple applications
                       No thermal Injury
- Low cost, reusable rigid and semi-rigid probes (0.8 ~ 3.2 mm)

Combination lithotripsy

- Combination of both ultrasonic and pneumatic
- Ultrasonic is better (12.9 mins to clear stone) than pneumatic (23.4 mins to clear stone)
- But combination lithotripsy is better than that (7.4 mins to clear stone).
- (Auge, 2002)

3.6   The Nephrostomy vs. Stent Debate Post PCNL

The routine use of the nephrostomy tube after PCNL has been subsequently questioned (Hüsch, 2015). Currently, the nephrostomy tube is increasingly omitted, and the access tract can be sealed by haemostatic agents (Hüsch, 2015). A ureteric stent is commonly inserted at the end of the procedure (Hüsch, 2015). However, the application of haemostatic sealants increases the immediate costs significantly (Hüsch, 2015).

The current body of literature does not provide high-level evidence for the preferred treatment of the access tract in PCNL (Hüsch, 2015).

References

Kalogeropoulou C, Kallidonis P, Liatsikos EN. Imaging in percutaneous Nephrolithotomy. J Endourol. 2009 Oct;23(10):1571–7.

Zeng GH, Liu Y, Zhong W, Fei X, Song Y. The role of middle calyx puncture in percutaneous nephrolithotomy: relative factors and choice considerations. Minerva Urol Nefrol. 2015 Dec;67(4):335–45.

Rivera M, Viers B, Cockerill P, Agarwal D, Mehta R, Krambeck A. Pre- and postoperative predictors of infection-related complications in patients undergoing percutaneous Nephrolithotomy. J Endourol. 2016 Sep;30(9):982–6.

Patel RM, Okhunov Z, Clayman RV, Landman J. Prone versus supine percutaneous Nephrolithotomy: what is your position? Curr Urol Rep. 2017 Apr;18(4):26.

Kim SC, Tinmouth WW, Kuo RL, Paterson RF, Lingeman JE. Using and choosing a tube after percutaneous nephrolithotomy for large or complex stone disease: a treatment strategy. J Endourol. 2005 Apr;19(3):348–52.

Auge BK, Preminger GM. Update on shock wave lithotripsy technology. Curr Opin Urol. 2002 Jul;12(4):287–90.

Hüsch T, Reiter M, Mager R, Steiner E, Herrmann TRW, Haferkamp A, Schilling D. The Management of the Access Tract after Percutaneous Nephrolithotomy. World J Urol. 2015;33(12):1921–8.

Management of PCNL Complications

4

4.1 Bleeding Post PCNL- Risk Factors and Steps in Management

PCNL
- An often aggressive procedure, requiring puncture into a renal calyx
- Uses a variety of techniques including a nephroscope, different types of lithotripsy, and often single or multiple puncture techniques
- As part of the puncture process, on either side, the spleen, liver, adjacent viscera can be damaged.
- Immediate or delayed bleeding can also occur.

Bleeding post operatively
- Can be heavy, depending upon the location of the puncture- if close to vessels, the surgeon must be very careful when placing the puncture
- Anatomy must always be key when placing a puncture, with scans reviewed beforehand
- Most haemorrhage occurs from the renal parenchyma
- The Transfusion rate is approximately 7% (Kriazis 2015)
- The access sheath provides intra-operative tamponade of parenchymal bleeding

Risk factors for bleeding
- Multiple punctures, more common in USA, give a higher risk of bleeding
- Increasing tract size will also have more bleeding- less likely with mini and ultramini PCNL
- Alkan dilators more likely to bleed, as compared to balloon dilators
- Prolonged procedure with more extensive dissection time
- Renal pelvic perforation- area less likely to heal
- (Aghamir, 2016)

Steps to minimise bleeding
- Strictly puncture through a calyx
- Avoid the renal pelvis in punctures
- Minimal trauma to tract
- Use flexible scope for stones in other calyces, instead of multiple punctures

Management of bleeding
- Cauterization/suture to stop, if from tract
- Apply pressure to the incision
- Placement of Flowseal/ fibrillar
- Occlude the nephrostomy tube
- Kaye Nephrostomy Tamponade Balloon
- Rarely, embolisation, nephrectomy may happen
- (Ganpule, 2014)

4.2   Management of Delayed Bleeding

Delayed bleeding

- Occurs in <1%
- Causes can be Arteriovenous fistulas, Arterial
  pseudoaneurysms
- Bright red blood in the urine
- Angiography diagnostic in more than 90% of cases
- Selective angio-embolization is highly effective (success rate 94%)
- (Yamaguchi, 2011)

4.3   Management of Sepsis Post PCNL

Sepsis post PCNL
<30% of pts have fever post PCNL; most do not have an
infection
- Sepsis occurs in 1-2%
- When sepsis does occur, it must be treated quickly

- **Risk factors for fever include**
- Pre-operative urinary tract infection, some persist despite
  treatment- urine sample for microscopy is key
- Infectious stones - magnesium- ammonium- phosphate stones
- Poor drainage or obstruction
- Indwelling ureteric stent
- Nephrostomy tube

Treatment
- Treatment must be focused around culture results
- If infection pre-op, treat with culture-specific antibiotics, then
  discuss with microbiology lab and alter antibiotics if needed
- If obstructed, unobstruct the urinary system
- Try and keep irrigation pressure < 30mmhg
- If puss aspirated when creating tract, safest to place nephrostomy
  tube, admit and treat for sepsis, and delay surgical procedure.

4.4   Renal/Collecting System Injury Post PCNL

Collecting system injury

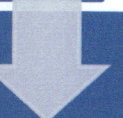

- Can occur during initial access or during dilation or lithotripsy.
- If noted intra-operatively, abort the procedure unless nearly complete.
- Collapse of a previously distended renal pelvis is the usual sign.
- Place nephrostomy plus ureteral stent to optimize drainage
- If missed intra-operatively might be heralded by postoperative abdominal distension, ileus, and/or fever
- Nephrostogram at 1-2 weeks.

4.5   Injury to Adjacent Viscera

Injury to adjacent viscera

Any abdominal organ close to the kidney can be injured

Pleura, colon, duodenum, jejunum, spleen, liver, and biliary system

Colon injury occurs at a rate of less than 1% / pleural injury 0-5%

Left colon injured twice as often (USS can reduce risk)

Additional risk factors include

Elderly- have large floppy colons

Dilated colon, due to bowel obstruction

Prior colon surgery or disease

Thin body patient

Horseshoe kidney

Injury might be less likely in the supine position

Most extraperitoneal and can be managed conservatively

The main principle of care: prompt and separate drainage of the colon and urinary collecting system

4.6   Outcomes in PCNL-Complications and Risk Factors

Kumar assesed complications based on CCS and predicted risk factors across the entire cohort and individually for pediatric (P: ≤18 years), adult (A: 19-65 years) and geriatric (G: ≥65 years) subgroups to assess the risk factors in each subset (Kumar, 2017)

Out of 922 (P=61; A=794; G=67) PCNL, 259 (28.09%) complications occurred with CCS I, II, III and IV constituting 152 (16.49%), 72 (7.81%), 31 (3.36%) and 4 (0.43%) respectively and its distribution was similar across the subsets and majority (224; 24.3%) were minor (CCS-1, 2) (Kumar, 2017). Placement of a nephrostomy (47.4%; 18/38) in Group P, supracostal access,≥2 punctures, higher GSS, nephrostomy, staghorn stones, ≥2 stones, stone size in Group A and hydronephrosis and prolonged OT in Group G were significantly associated with complications (Kumar, 2017).

On logistic regression, need of nephrostomy (adj. OR - 4.549), OT (adj. OR - 1.364) and supracostal access (adj. OR - 1.471) significantly contributed to complications in the study population. LOH was found to be significantly associated with complications (p<0.001) (Kumar, 2017). Contrary to the belief that extremes of ages are associated with complications of prone PCNL, we found age does not alter the incidence or grade of complications and LOH (Kumar, 2017).

References

Kyriazis I, Panagopoulos V, Kallidonis P, Özsoy M, Vasilas M, Liatsikos E. Complications in percutaneous nephrolithotomy. World J Urol. 2015 Aug;33(8):1069–77.

Aghamir SM, Elmimehr R, Modaresi SS, Salavati A. Comparing bleeding complications of double and single access totally tubeless PCNL: is it safe to obtain more accesses? Urol Int. 2016;96(1):73–6.

Ganpule AP, Shah DH, Desai MR. Postpercutaneous nephrolithotomy bleeding: aetiology and management. Curr Opin Urol. 2014 Mar;24(2):189–94.

Yamaguchi A, Skolarikos A, Buchholz NP, Chomón GB, Grasso M, Saba P, Nakada S, de la Rosette J. Clinical research office of the Endourological society percutaneous Nephrolithotomy study group. Operating times and bleeding complications in percutaneous nephrolithotomy: a comparison of tract dilation methods in 5,537 patients in the clinical research office of the Endourological society percutaneous Nephrolithotomy global study. J Endourol. 2011 Jun;25(6):933–9.

Kumar S, Keshavamurthy R, Karthikeyan VS, Mallya A. Complications after prone PCNL in pediatric, adult and geriatric patients – a single center experience over 7 years. Int Braz J Urol. 2017;43(4):704–12.

Types of Lithotripsy for PCNL

5.1 Types of Lithotripsy: Ultrasonic, Pneumatic or Combination

Types of Lithotripsy
- Extracorporeal
- Intracorporeal
- Ultrasonic
- Pneumatic

Ultrasonic lithotripsy
- First described to fragment renal calculi in 1979
- Hollow probe (2.5 ~ 4 F)
  Has advantage of "vacuum" capabilities
- High frequency (> 20 kHz) mechanical vibration generated by piezoelectric transducers
- "Drilling and grinding" of the target stone (Figs. 5.1 and 5.2)

Pneumatic lithotripsy
- Pneumatically driven piston fragments stones by direct contact
- Major advantages: Improved efficacy
  Multiple applications
  No thermal Injury
- Low cost, reusable rigid and semi-rigid probes (0.8 ~ 3.2 mm) (Figs. 5.3 and 5.4)

Combination lithotripsy
- Combination of both ultrasonic and pneumatic (Figure 5)
- Ultrasonic is better (12.9 mins to clear stone) than pneumatic (23.4 mins to clear stone)
- But combination lithotripsy is better than that (7.4 mins to clear stone).
- (Auge, 2002)

S. S. Goonewardene et al., *Surgical Strategies in Endourology for Stone Disease*, https://doi.org/10.1007/978-3-030-82143-2_5

Fig. 5.1 Ultrasonic
Lithotripsy

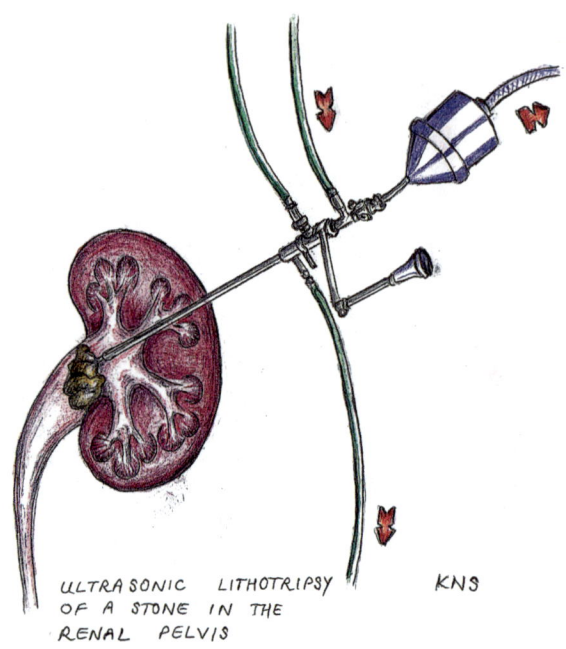

ULTRASONIC   LITHOTRIPSY   KNS
OF A STONE IN THE
RENAL   PELVIS

Fig. 5.2 Components of
an Ultrasonic Lithotripter

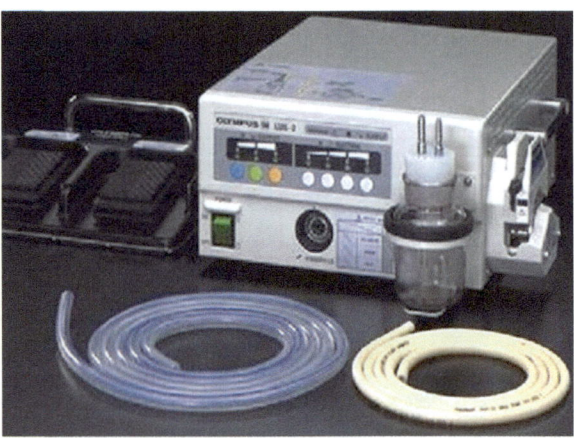

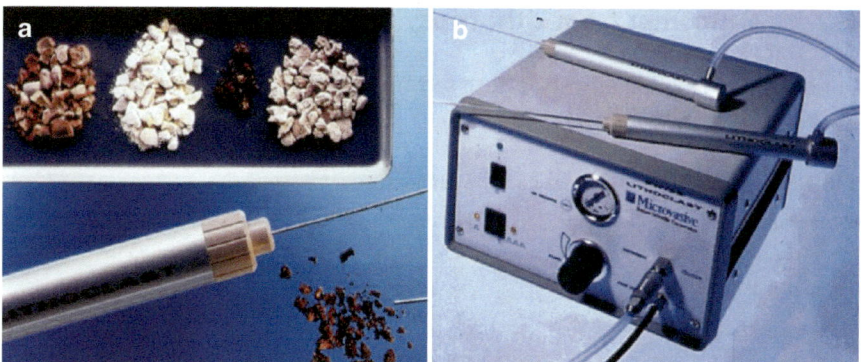

Fig. 5.3 (**a** and **b**) Pneumatic Lithotripsy

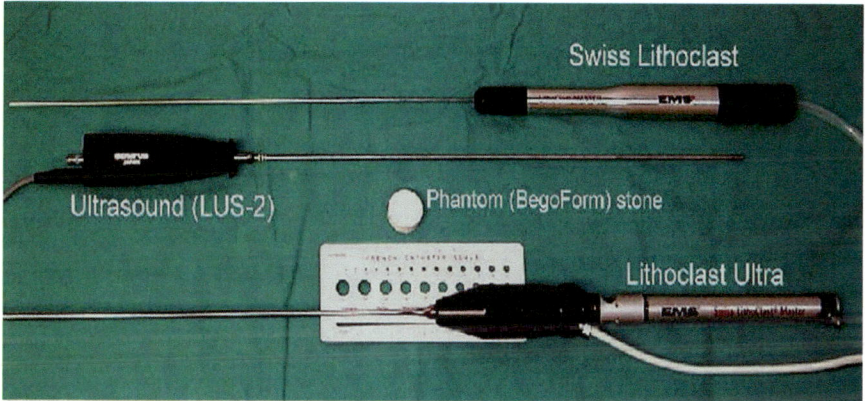

Fig. 5.4 Combination Lithotripsy

5.2   Outcomes from Lithotripsy

For outcomes from lithotripsty, please see Tables 5.1 and 5.2.

Table 5.1 Stone free rates during shockwave lithotripsy

Stone size	<1 cm	1–2 cm	2–3 cm	>3 cm
% Stone free	95%	87%	48%	35%

Lingeman et al. (1990)

Table 5.2 Fragmentation Results from Lithotripsy

	Pneumatic	Ultrasound	Combination
Average size of fragments (mm)	9.1	3.7 (p < 0.0001)	1.7 (p < 0.0001)
Time to fragment clearance (min)	23.8	12.9 (<0.003)	7.4 (<0.003)

Auge and Preminger (2002)

References

Auge BK, Preminger GM. Update on shock wave lithotripsy technology. Curr Opin Urol. 2002 Jul;12(4):287–90.

Lingeman JE, Woods JR, Toth PD. Blood pressure changes following extracorporeal shock wave lithotripsy and other forms of treatment for nephrolithiasis. JAMA. 1990 Apr 4;263(13):1789–94.

PCNL Strategy for a Staghorn Stone

6

6.1 Guidelines on Staghorn Stones

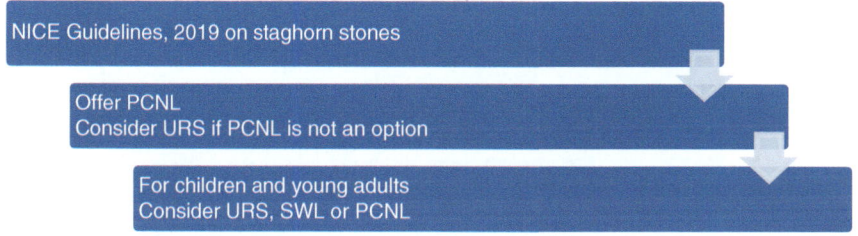

NICE Guidelines 2019 on Stones.

S. S. Goonewardene et al., *Surgical Strategies in Endourology for Stone Disease*,
https://doi.org/10.1007/978-3-030-82143-2_6

6.2   Management of Staghorn Stones and Related Outcomes

An aggressive approach to staghorns (Blandy, 1976)

Treatment vs. conservative management of a large staghorn stone in situ in 60 cases is compared to the risk of operative removal in 125 cases (Blandy, 1976). The overall mortality rate in patients treated conservatively was 28 percent, carcinoma developing in 4 cases and a life-threatening pyonephrosis in 16 (Blandy, 1976). Of patients treated by removal of the stone the mortality rate was 7.2 percent (during 10 years of observation) and stones recurred in 21 cases (Blandy, 1976). These studies refute the notion of the silent staghorn calculus and demonstrate that operative removal is safer for the patient and kidney (Blandy, 1976).

In the 17 years up to 1979 189 kidneys have had an extended pyelolithotomy for staghorn calculus and have been followed up (Woodhouse, 1981). In only 1 of 96 unilateral cases did a stone form in a normal contralateral kidney, whatever the outcome of surgery on the affected side (Woodhouse, 1981). Seven early nephrectomies were performed for non-function and in 6 bilateral cases, with advanced renal failure, surgery did not arrest the loss of renal function (Woodhouse, 1981).

Regrowth of stone occurred in 43 cases (complete staghorns in 24). Regrowth did not occur in 18 of 20 incompletely cleared kidneys nor in 22 of 41 with persistent infection (Woodhouse, 1981). Renal function was improved in 13 of 15 cases where it had not already deteriorated beyond a critical point (Woodhouse, 1981). It is concluded that unilateral staghorn stones may be treated in their own right, without fear of compromising a normal contralateral kidney; that regrowth of stones is not inevitable, even with incomplete clearance; and that renal function is usually improved by surgery (Woodhouse, 1981).

6.3   Case 1 Fragmentation of Staghorn Stone and Forceps Removal

The case

- 54 year old female
- Recurrent UTIs
- Chronic right sided pain for months

The condition

- Right-sided staghorn stone

Pre-operative imaging and strategy

- X ray KUB
- Allows debulking of large stones
- (Should push PNL "to the limit")
- SWL reserved for inaccessible fragments
- Flexible nephroscopyto ensure stone-free status (Figs. 6.1, 6.2 and Table 6.1)

The equipment

- Rigid cystoscopy, ureteric balloon catheter and sensor wire
- Rigid nephroscope
- Flexible nephroscope
- Ultrasonic device
- Pneumatic device
- Flexible ureteroscope

The strategy

- Rigid cystoscope in, with bridge
- Ureteric catheter up, with sensor, retrograde and occlude ureter
- Place puncture in a position to clear the majority of stone with one puncture.
- Fragment and extract, if necessary switch to flexible ureteroscopy and holmium laser.
- 6x24 fr stent, nephrostomy.

The difficulties

- Placing a puncture that adequately clears all stone fragments.
- Risk of vascular injury.
- Properly clearing stone, which may be in a dependant position.
- Additionally, the flexible ureteroscope may have to be used with a holmium laser or bipolar forceps to extract stone.
- Try and avoid a 2nd operation (Diri, 2018)

The outcome

- Stones fully cleared from kidney.
- Chase stone type.
- Stent register-tract stent and ensure it is removed.
- Dietary advice including BAUS information leaflet.
- TFTs, Calcium, Urate

Fig. 6.1 Xray KUB
demonstrating right sided
staghorn stone

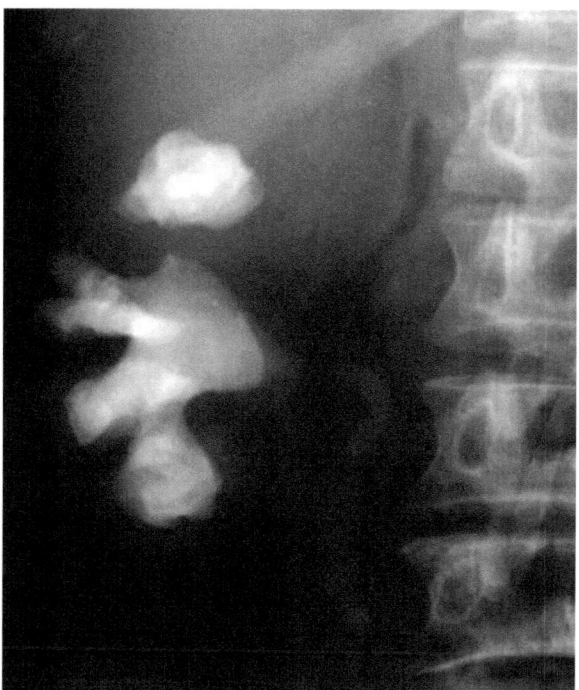

Fig. 6.2 Retrieving stone
fragments using a flexible
Ureteroscope

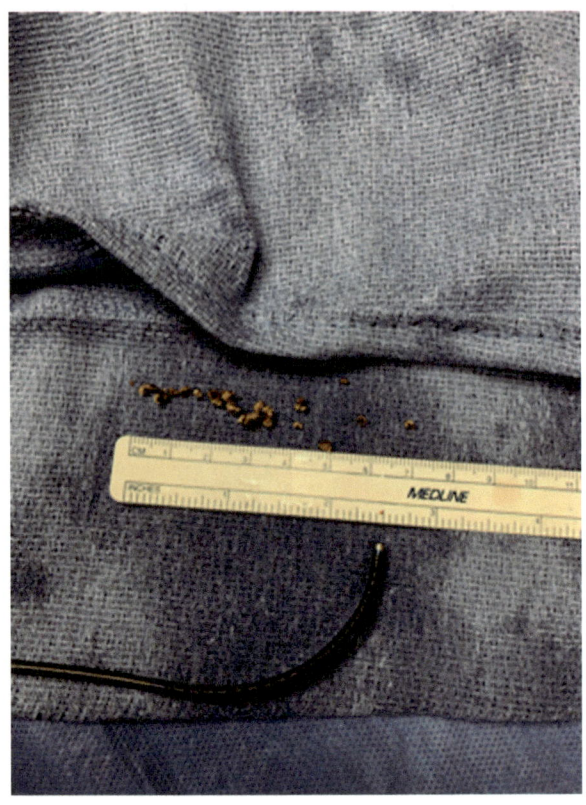

Table 6.1 Stone free rates with staghorn calculi

	SWL	PCNL	Comination therapy	Open Surgery
% stone free rate	50%	73%	81%	82%

Türk et al. (2008)

6.4   Case 2 the Multiple Puncture for a Staghorn Stone

The case
- 55 year old male
- Recurrent UTIs
- Bilateral loin pain for months

The condition
- Bilateral staghorn stones

Pre-operative imaging
- X ray KUB (Figs. 6.3, 6.4, 6.5, 6.6, 6.7 and 6.8 for preoperative imaging and introperative imaging)

Fig. 6.3 Xray KUB demonstrating bilateral staghorn stones

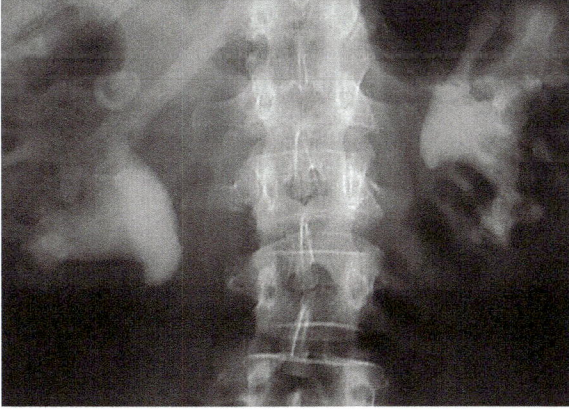

Fig. 6.4 Pre-
operative IVU

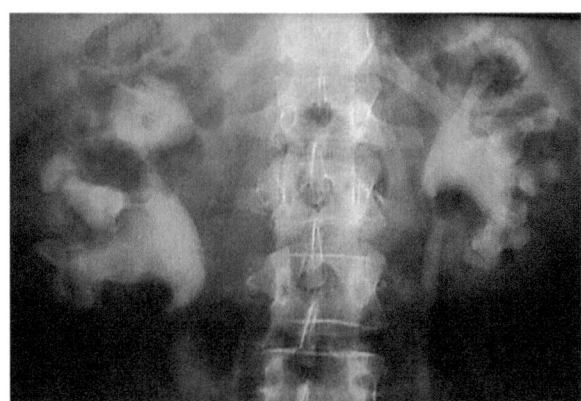

Fig. 6.5 Fluoroscopy
demonstrating multiple
puncture access with
guidewires passed

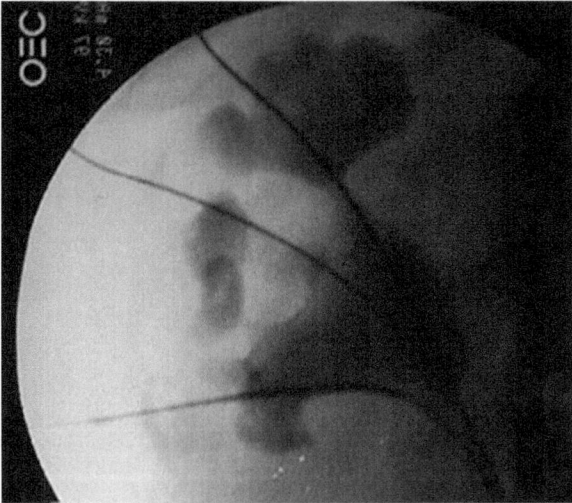

Fig. 6.6 3 access sheaths
inserted as part of a
multipuncture approach

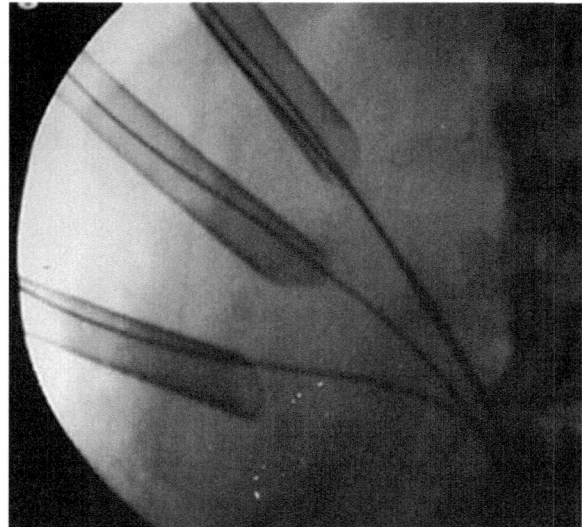

Fig. 6.7 Clearing the
upper pole of stone Using
a Nephroscope

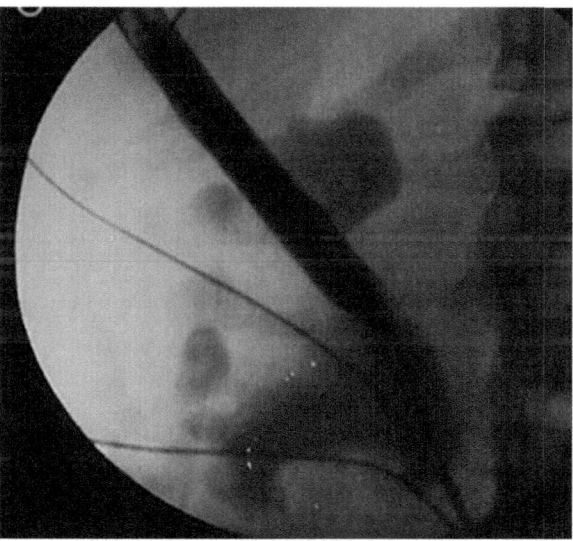

Fig. 6.8 3 Nephrostomy
tubes inserted

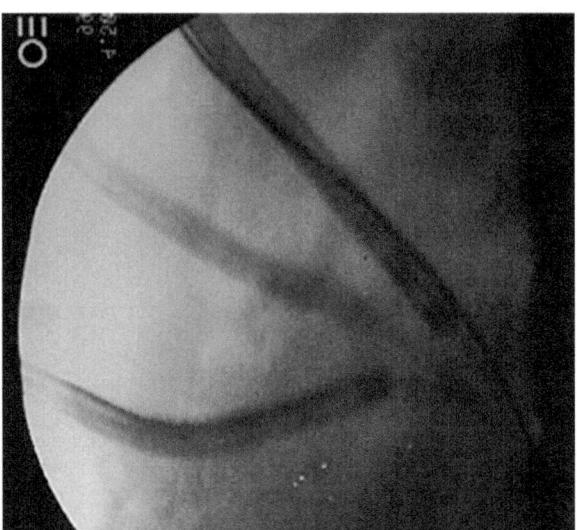

The equipment

- Rigid cystoscopy, ureteric balloon catheter and sensor wire
- Rigid nephroscope
- Flexible nephroscope
- Ultrasonic device
- Pneumatic device
- Flexible ureteroscope

The strategy

- Rigid cystoscope in, with bridge
- Ureteric catheter up, with sensor, retrograde and occlude ureter
- Usually, most PCNLs, we try to do with one puncture-this case requires multiple.
- Fragment and extract, if necessary switch to flexible ureteroscopy and holmium laser.
- 6x24 fr stent, nephrstomies

The difficulties

- The right side was managed 1st
- Placing a puncture that adequately clears all stone fragments-more than one puncture is required.
- Risk of vascular injury and also chest or bowel injury.
- Properly clearing stone, which may be in a dependant position.
- Additionally, the flexible ureteroscope may have to be used with a holmium laser or bipolar forceps to extract stone.

The outcome

- Do not fear upper pole access
- Command rigid and flexible nephroscopy
- Command several lithotripsy options
- The right side was completely cleared.
- The left side is waiting to be treated (case 3)

6.5   Case 3 Sandwich Therapy for a Left-Sided Stone

The case
- 55 male
- Recurrent UTIS
- Bilateral loin pain for months

The condition
- Bilateral staghorn stones
- Right side treated in case 2
- Left stag horn left behind

Pre- operative imaging and strategy
- X ray KUB (Figs. 6.9 and 6.10)
- Day 1:PNL to debulk at least 90% of stone
- Day 3:SWL for remaining fragments
- Day 5:Flex / rigid nephroscopy to remove any residual remnants. Inspect each calyx
- Nephrostomy tube not replaced

The equipment

- Rigid cystoscopy, ureteric balloon catheter and sensor wire
- Rigid nephroscope
- Flexible nephroscope
- Ultrasonic device
- Pneumatic device
- Flexible ureteroscope
- Extracorporeal ESWL

The strategy

- Rigid cystoscope in, with bridge
- Ureteric catheter up, with sensor, retrograde and occlude ureter
- Usually, most PCNLs, we try to do with one puncture-this case requires multiple.
- Fragment and extract, if necessary switch to flexible ureteroscopy and holmiumn laser.
- 6x24 fr stent, nephrstomies

The difficulties

- PNL Allows debulking of large stones
    (Should push PNL "to the limit")
- SWL reserved for inaccessible fragments
- Flexible nephroscopy to ensure stone-free status

The outcome

- Do not fear upper pole access
- Command rigid and flexible nephroscopy
- Command several lithotripsy options
- The right side was completely cleared.
- The left side is waiting to be treated (case 3)

Fig. 6.9 Xray KUB
demonstrating a left
staghorn stone

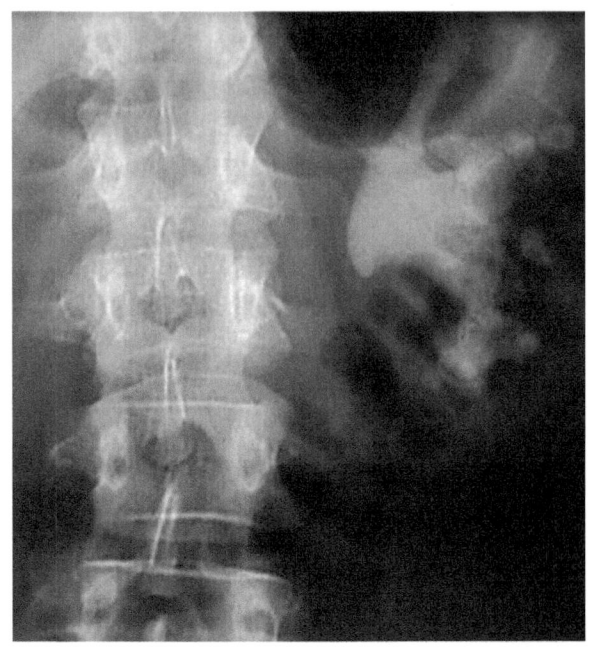

Fig. 6.10 Demonstrating
the IVU

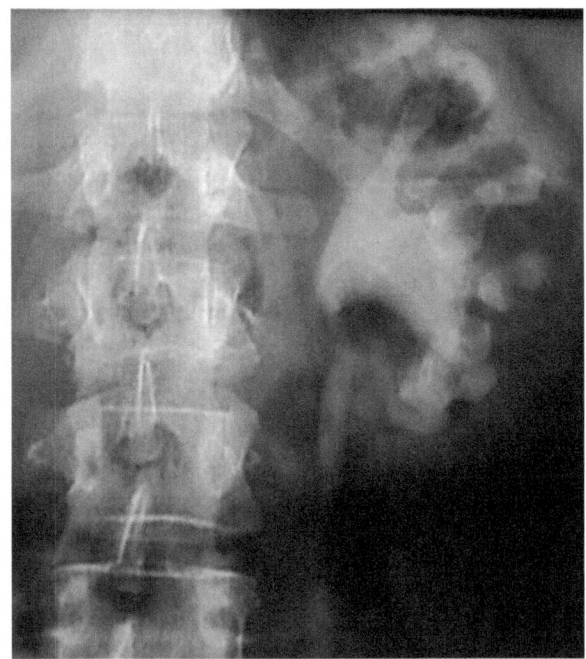

References

Blandy JP, Singh M. The case for a more aggressive approach to staghorn stones. J Urol. 1976;115(5):505–6.

Diri A, Diri B. Management of staghorn renal stones. Ren Fail. 2018 Nov;40(1):357–62.

NICE. Guideline - renal and ureteric stones: assessment and management: NICE (2019) renal and ureteric stones: assessment and management. BJU Int. 2019 Feb;123(2):220–32.

Türk C, Knoll T, Köhrmann KU. New guidelines for urinary stone treatment. Controversy or development? Urologe A. 2008 May;47(5):591–3.

Woodhouse CR, Farrell CR, Paris AM, Blandy JP. The place of extended Pyelolithotomy (Gil-Vernet operation) in the management of renal staghorn calculi. Br J Urol. 1981;53(6):520–3.

PCNL Strategy for Lower Calyceal Stones

7.1 Guidelines for Staghorn Stones

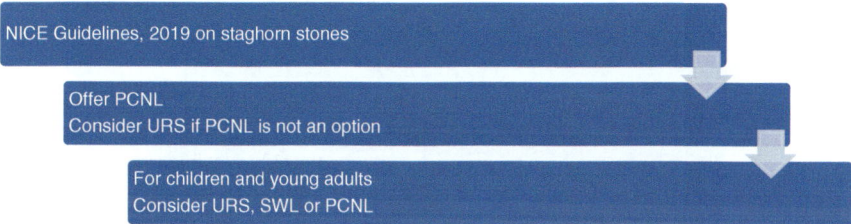

NICE Guidelines (2019).

7.2   Supine Vs. Prone PCNL Outcomes

Sanguedolce assessed efficacy and safety of prone- and supine percutaneous nephrolithotomy (PCNL) for the treatment of lower pole kidney stones (Sanguedolce, 2013). One hundred seventeen patients underwent PCNL (mean stone size: 19.5 mm) for stones harboured only in the lower renal pole (single stone: 53.6%; multiple stones: 46.4%) (Sanguedolce, 2013). A higher proportion of patients with ASA score ≥ 3 and harbouring multiple lower pole stones were treated with supine PCNL (5.8 vs. 23.1%; p = 0.0001, and 25 vs. 81.5%; p = 0.0001, respectively, for prone- and supine PCNL) (Sanguedolce, 2013).

One-month SFR was 88.9%; an auxiliary procedure was needed in 6 patients; the 3-month SFR was 90.2% (Sanguedolce, 2013). There were 9 post-operative major complications (7.7%). No differences were observed in terms of 1- and 3-month SFRs (90.4 vs. 87.7%; p = 0.64; 92.3 vs. 89.2%; p = 0.4) and complication rates (7.6 vs. 7.7%; p = 0.83) when comparing prone- versus supine PCNL, respectively (Sanguedolce, 2013).

The results confirm the high success rate and relatively low morbidity of modern PCNL for lower pole stones, regardless the position used (Sanguedolce, 2013). Supine PCNL was more frequently offered in case of patients with higher ASA score and in case of multiple lower pole stones (Sanguedolce, 2013).

7.3 Case 1 PCNL for Multiple Stones Within the Lower Pole

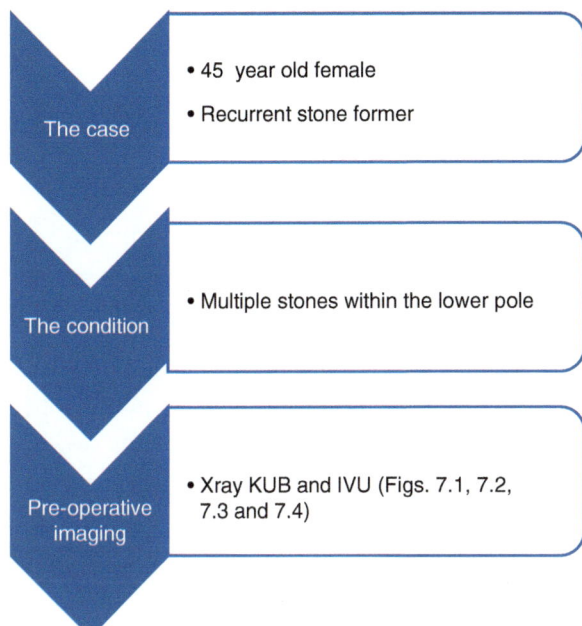

The case
- 45 year old female
- Recurrent stone former

The condition
- Multiple stones within the lower pole

Pre-operative imaging
- Xray KUB and IVU (Figs. 7.1, 7.2, 7.3 and 7.4)

Fig. 7.1 Xray KUB-
stones in the lower pole

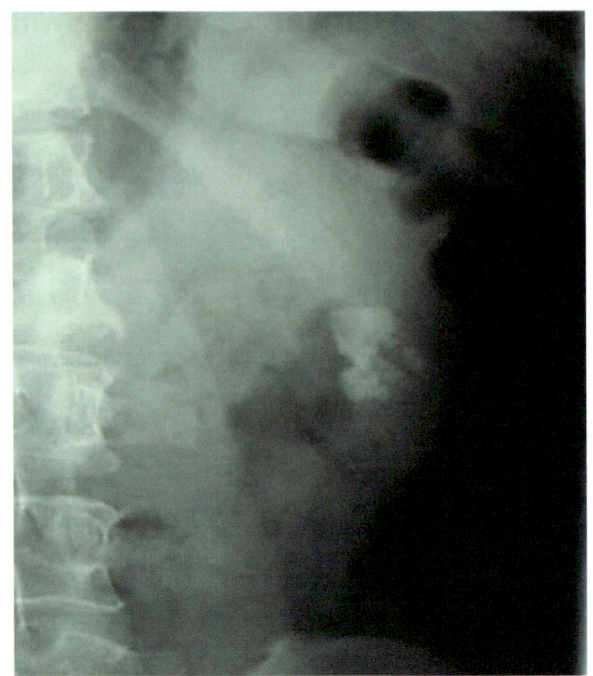

Fig. 7.2 IVU
demonstrating drainage

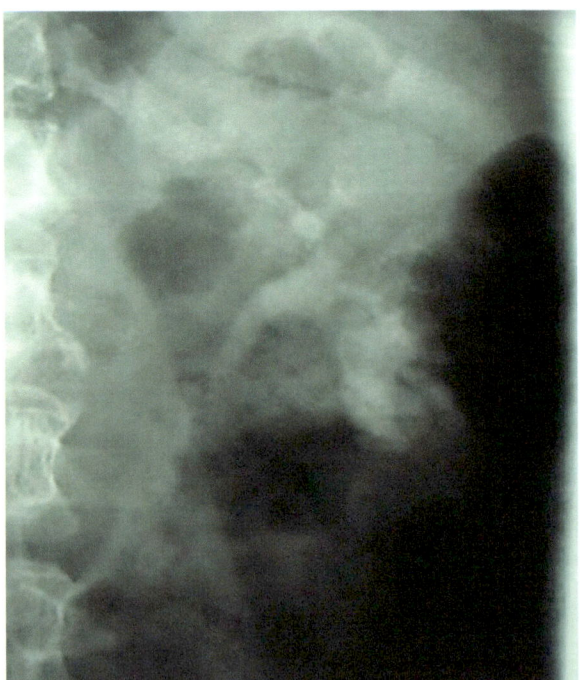

Fig. 7.3 Puncture into the
lower pole calyx

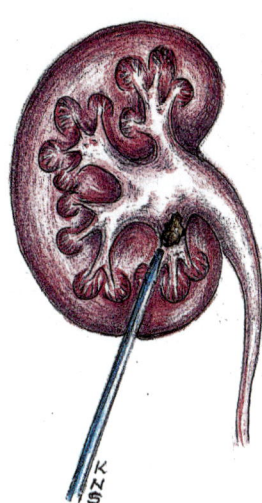

PUNCTURE   INTO   THE
LOWER   POLE   CALYX
TO   PLACE   A   STENT
OR   NEPHROSTOMY   TUBE

Fig. 7.4 Puncture onto a lower pole stone

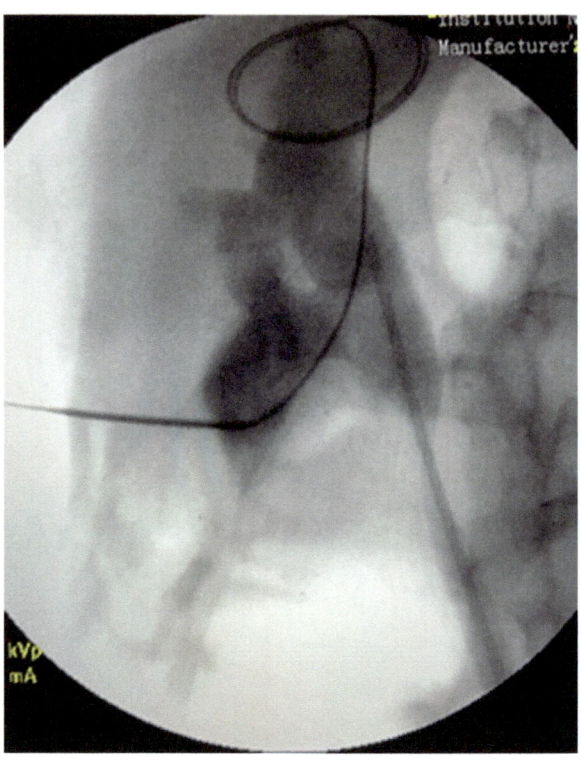

The equipment

- Sensor wire 0.08 Fr- nitinol core over a hydrophilic coating
- Ureteric balloon catheter
- Contrast- Urograffin 150 or 300.
- Rigid nephroscope
- Flexible nephroscope
- Ultrasonic device
- Pneumatic device
- Flexible ureteroscope

The strategy

- Rigid cystoscope in, with bridge
- Do cystoscopy and retrograde study
- Place ureteric balloon catheter
- Identify stones with fluoroscopy, or us
- Using Seldinger technique, place tract and perc onto stone
- Using nephroscope fragment stone and extract
- Place nephrostomy and stent

The difficulties

- Piercing onto the stone without injuring adjacent viscera
- A subcostal approach must be taken for lower pole stones, so this risk is higher.
- Stone must be repositioned in the midpole calyx, this is a better position for fragmentation
- Properly clearing stone, which may be in a dependant position.
- Rate of vascular injury is higher in lower pole stone compared to mid calyceal stone
- PCNL does give better stone clearance rates than ESWL (Bozzini, 2017)

The outcome

- Stones fully cleared from the kidney.
- Chase stone type.
- Stent register- tract stent and ensure it is removed.
- Dietary advice including BAUS information leaflet.
- TFTs, Calcium, Urate.

7.4   To Stent or Place a Nephrostomy Tube Post PCNL- the Debate

To stent or place a Nephrostomy tube post PCNL

• EAU Guidelines 2019

The decision on whether, or not, to place a nephrostomy tube at the conclusion of the PNL procedure depends on several factors, including:

-presence of residual stones;

-likelihood of a second-look procedure;

-significant intra-operative blood loss;

-urine extravasation;

-ureteral obstruction;

-potential persistent bacteriuria due to infected stones;

-solitary kidney;

-bleeding diathesis;

-planned percutaneous chemolitholysis.

7.5   Optimal Management of Lower Calyceal Stones

The optimal management of lower calyceal stones is still controversial because no single method is suitable for the removal of all lower calyceal stones (Yuri, 2018). Minimally invasive procedures such as extracorporeal shock wave lithotripsy (ESWL), percutaneous nephrolithotomy (PCNL) and flexible ureteroscopy (fURS) are the therapeutic methods for lower calyceal stones (Yuri, 2018).

The stone free rate from 958 patients (271 PCNL, 174 fURS and 513 ESWL), 3 months after operation, was 90.8% (246/271) after PCNL; 75.3% (131/174) after fURS; and 64.7% (332/513) after ESWL (Yuri, 2018). Base on stone free rate in 10-20 mm lower pole stone following management, PCNL is better than fURS (overall RR was 1.32 (95% CI 1.13 - 1.55); p<0.001 and I2=57%) and ESWL (overall risk ratio 1.42 (95% CI 1.30 - 1.55); p=<0.001 and I2 = 85%) (Yuri, 2018).

FURS is better than ESWL on stone free rate in 10-20 mm lower pole stone management with overall RR 1.16 (95% CI 1.04 - 1.30; p=0.01 and I2=40%) (Yuri, 2018).

References

Bozzini G, Verze P, Arcaniolo D, Dal Piaz O, Buffi NM, Guazzoni G, Provenzano M, Osmolorskij B, Sanguedolce F, Montanari E, Macchione N, Pummer K, Mirone V, De Sio M, Taverna G. A prospective randomized comparison among SWL, PCNL and RIRS for lower calyceal stones less than 2 cm: a multicenter experience : a better understanding on the treatment options for lower pole stones. World J Urol. 2017 Dec;35(12):1967–75.

NICE Guideline. Renal and ureteric stones: assessment and management: NICE (2019) renal and ureteric stones: assessment and management. BJU Int. 2019 Feb;123(2):220–32.

Sanguedolce F, Breda A, Millan F, Brehmer M, Knoll T, Liatsikos E, Osther P, Traxer O, Scoffone C. Lower pole stones: prone PCNL versus supine PCNL in the International Cooperation in Endourology (ICE) group experience world. J Urol. 2013;31(6):1575–80.

Türk C, et al. EAU guidelines on interventional treatment for urolithiasis. Eur Urol. 2016 March;69(3):475–82.

Yuri P, Hariwibowo R, Soeroharjo I, Danarto R, Hendri AZ, Brodjonegoro SR, Rasyid N, Birowo P, Widyahening IS. Meta-analysis of optimal management of lower pole stone of 10–20 mm: Flexible Ureteroscopy (FURS) Versus Extracorporeal Shock Wave Lithotripsy (ESWL) Versus Percutaneus Nephrolithotomy (PCNL). Acta Med Indones. 2018;50(1):18–25.

PCNL Strategy for Upper Calyceal Stones

8

8.1 Guidelines on Staghorn Stones

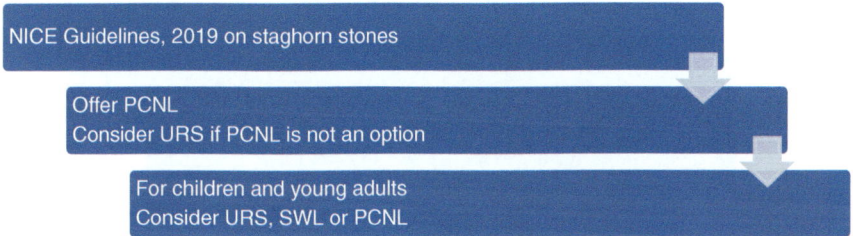

NICE Guidelines (2019) on renal stones.

S. S. Goonewardene et al., *Surgical Strategies in Endourology for Stone Disease*, https://doi.org/10.1007/978-3-030-82143-2_8

8.2   Outcomes of PCNL with Upper Calyceal Access

Tefelki, 2013 analyzed the indications for and outcomes of percutaneous nephrolithotomy using upper pole access (Tefelki, 2013).

The Clinical Research Office of the Endourological Society (CROES) assessed consecutive patients at 96 centres globally. Data on 4,494 patients were included (Tefelki, 2013). The upper pole access group had more staghorn stones (21.7% vs 15.5%, p <0.001) and a greater stone burden (mean ± SD 476 ± 390.5 vs 442 ± 344.9 mm(2), p = 0.091) (Tefelki, 2013). The stone-free rate was lower in the upper pole access group (77.1% vs 81.6%, p = 0.030) (Tefelki, 2013).

The overall complication rate was higher in the upper pole group with a higher incidence of hydrothorax (5.8% vs 1.5%) but a lower incidence of pelvic perforation (1.8% vs 3.2%) (Tefelki, 2013). Mean hospital stay was longer in the upper pole group (p = 0.048). Success and complication rates were similar in upper pole access subgroups, defined as definitive (staghorn and isolated upper calyceal stones) and elective (pelvic, middle calyceal and lower pole stones) indications (Tefelki, 2013).

Isolated upper pole access is indicated in a select group of patients with complex stones (Tefelki, 2013). Upper calyceal and staghorn stones are more commonly managed by upper pole access, which is associated with a higher complication rate and longer hospital stay as well as a lower stone-free rate due to procedure complexity (Tefelki, 2013).

8.3   PCNL Strategy for Upper Pole Stones

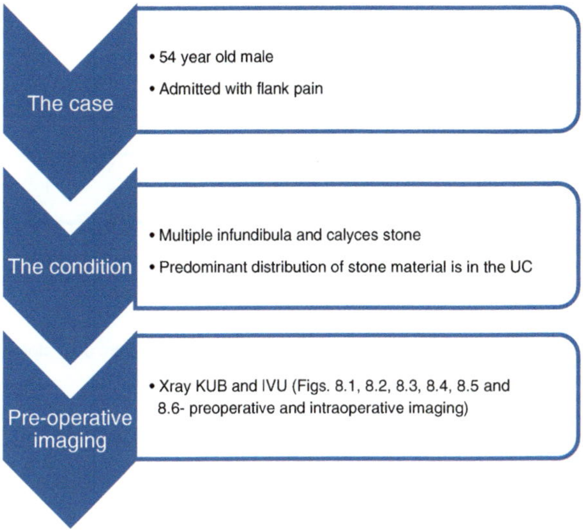

The case
- 54 year old male
- Admitted with flank pain

The condition
- Multiple infundibula and calyces stone
- Predominant distribution of stone material is in the UC

Pre-operative imaging
- Xray KUB and IVU (Figs. 8.1, 8.2, 8.3, 8.4, 8.5 and 8.6- preoperative and intraoperative imaging)

The equipment

- Sensor wire 0.08 Fr- nitinol core over a hydrophilic coating
- Ureteric balloon catheter
- Contrast- Urograffin 150 or 300.
- Rigid nephroscope
- Flexible nephroscope
- Ultrasonic device
- Pneumatic device
- Flexible ureteroscope

The strategy

- Rigid cystoscope in, with bridge
- Do cystoscopy and retrograde study
- Place ureteric balloon catheter
- Identify stones with fluoroscopy, or us
- Using seldinger technique, place tract and perc onto stone
- Using nephroscope fragment stone and extract
- Place nephrostomy and stent

The difficulties

- Piercing onto the stone without injuring adjacent viscera, 5% risk of hydropneumothorax (Patel, 2017)
- Properly clearing stone, which may require multiple punctures
- Rate of vascular injury is higher in lower pole stone compared to mid calyceal stone
- The overall complication rate was higher in the upper pole stones (Tefekli, 2013)

The outcome

- Stones fully cleared from kidney.
- Chase stone type.
- Stent register- tract stent and ensure it is removed.
- Dietary advice including BAUS information leaflet.
- TFTs, Calcium, Urate.

Fig. 8.1 Xray KUB
demonstrating stone

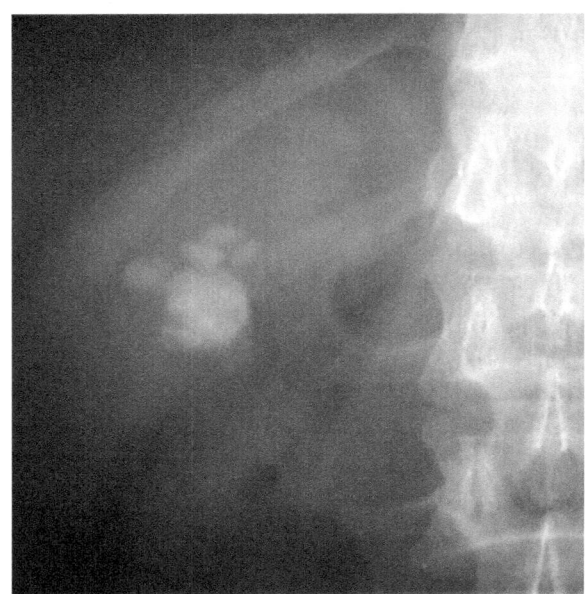

Fig. 8.2 IVU
demonstrating stone and
calyceal anatomy

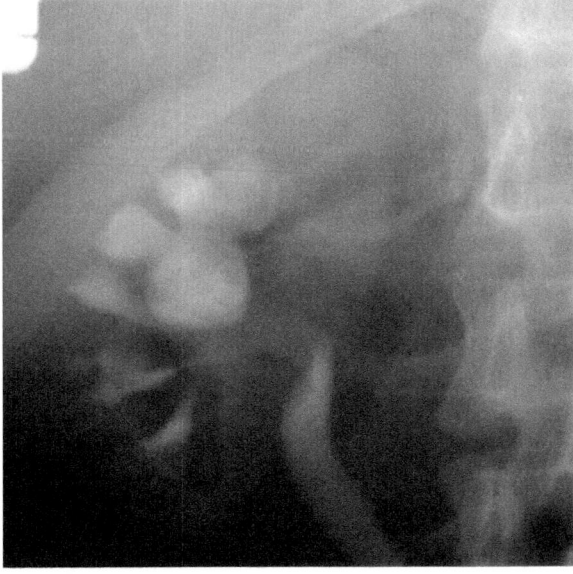

Fig. 8.3 Gaining access to the upper pole stone

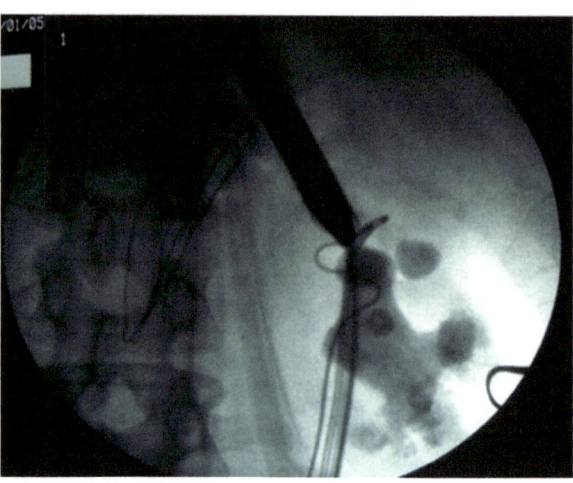

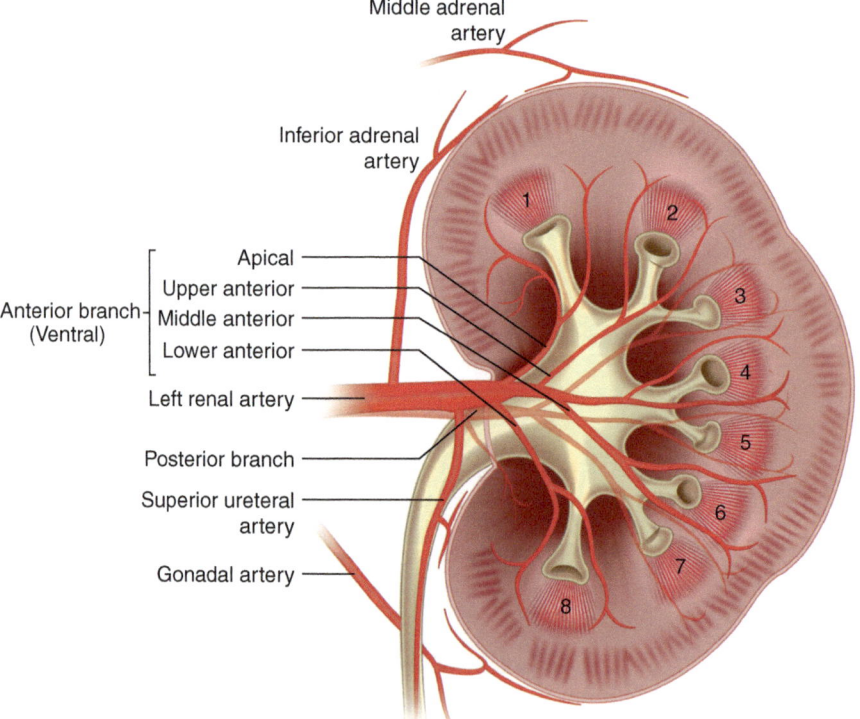

Fig. 8.4 Arterial supply to the kidney (Courtesy of David Albala)

Fig. 8.5 The ideal site for an upper pole puncture-into the tip of the calyx directly

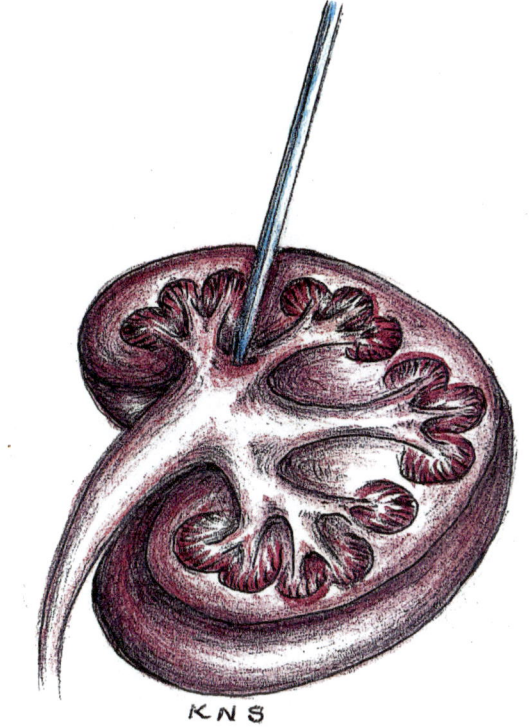

KNS

IDEAL SITE FOR
AN UPPER POLE PUNCTURE

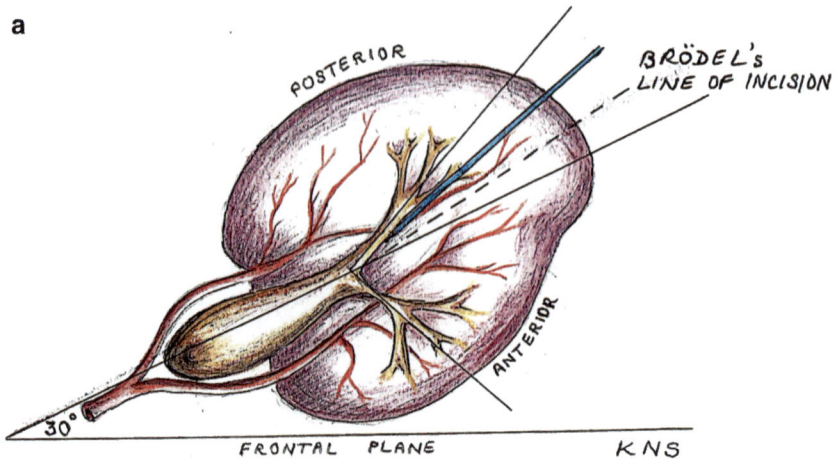

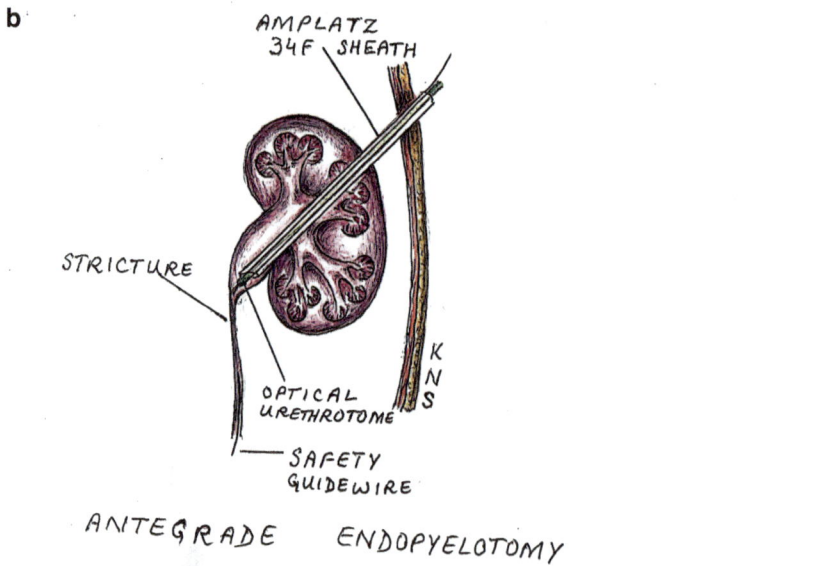

Fig. 8.6 (**a** and **b**) Demonstrating an upper pole posterior-lateral puncture

8.4   Impact of Renal Pelvic pressure on PCNL Outcome

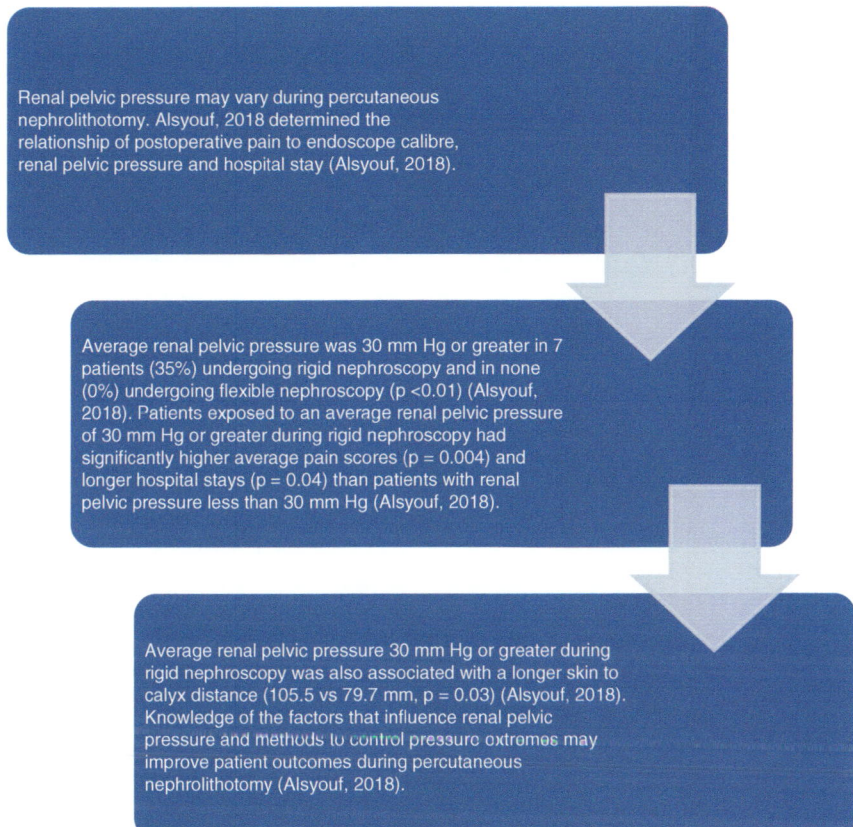

Renal pelvic pressure may vary during percutaneous nephrolithotomy. Alsyouf, 2018 determined the relationship of postoperative pain to endoscope calibre, renal pelvic pressure and hospital stay (Alsyouf, 2018).

Average renal pelvic pressure was 30 mm Hg or greater in 7 patients (35%) undergoing rigid nephroscopy and in none (0%) undergoing flexible nephroscopy (p <0.01) (Alsyouf, 2018). Patients exposed to an average renal pelvic pressure of 30 mm Hg or greater during rigid nephroscopy had significantly higher average pain scores (p = 0.004) and longer hospital stays (p = 0.04) than patients with renal pelvic pressure less than 30 mm Hg (Alsyouf, 2018).

Average renal pelvic pressure 30 mm Hg or greater during rigid nephroscopy was also associated with a longer skin to calyx distance (105.5 vs 79.7 mm, p = 0.03) (Alsyouf, 2018). Knowledge of the factors that influence renal pelvic pressure and methods to control pressure extremes may improve patient outcomes during percutaneous nephrolithotomy (Alsyouf, 2018).

References

Alsyouf M, Abourbih S, West B, Herbert H, Duane Baldwin D. Elevated renal pelvic pressures during percutaneous Nephrolithotomy risk higher postoperative pain and longer hospital stay. J Urol. 2018;199(1):193–9.

NICE Guideline. Renal and ureteric stones: assessment and management: NICE (2019) renal and ureteric stones: assessment and management. BJU Int. 2019 Feb;123(2):220–32.

Patel AP, Bui D, Pattaras J, Ogan K. Upper pole urologist-obtained percutaneous renal access for PCNL is safe and efficacious. Can J Urol. 2017 Apr;24(2):8754–8.

Tefekli A, Esen T, Olbert PJ, Tolley D, Nadler RB, Sun YH, Duvdevani M, de la Rosette JJ, CROES PCNL Study Group. Isolated upper pole access in percutaneous nephrolithotomy: a large-scale analysis from the CROES percutaneous nephrolithotomy global study. J Urol. 2013 Feb;189(2):568–73.

The Rigid Cystoscope

9

- Virtually all of the credit for the design of modern rod-lens endoscopes which has opened the door to modern "key-hole" surgery must be given to British Physicist Harold H. Hopkins (1918–1994). (Oxford Dictionary of National biography (online ed.). Oxford University Press 2004, doi https://doi.org/10.1093/ref:odnb/55032)
- Cystoscopy allows for direct visualization of the urethra, urethral sphincter, prostate, bladder and ureteral orifices as part of diagnostic procedures.
- The diameter of rigid cystoscopes varies between 6 F and 27 F; the most commonly used in adults having a diameter ranging between 15 F and 25 F (Akornor et al. 2005). In UK practice, this can vary between 17 and 22 fr.
- The modern rigid cystoscope is composed of four pieces: light source, telescope, bridge, and sheath (Fig. 9.1)

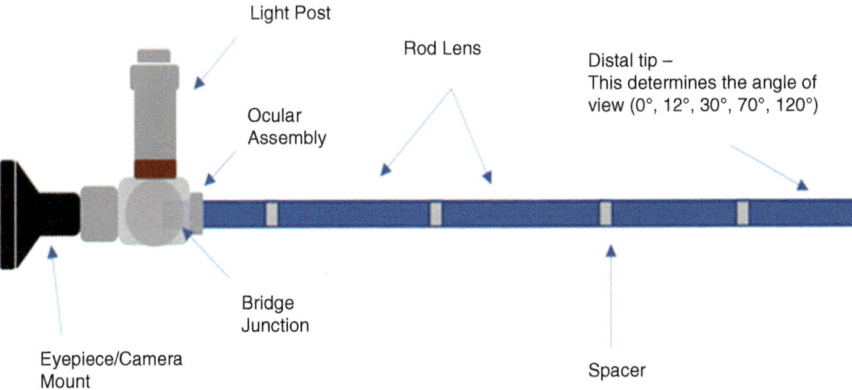

Light Post

Rod Lens

Distal tip –
This determines the angle of
view (0°, 12°, 30°, 70°, 120°)

Ocular
Assembly

Eyepiece/Camera
Mount

Bridge
Junction

Spacer

Fig. 9.1 The rod lens system of light refraction in a cystoscope. Image courtesy of Ms. Leveillee

© The Author(s), under exclusive license to Springer Nature
Switzerland AG 2021
S. S. Goonewardene et al., *Surgical Strategies in Endourology for Stone Disease*,
https://doi.org/10.1007/978-3-030-82143-2_9

In this system the air interface acts as the refractory agent.

Sometimes the sheath will come separately- the Albarran sheath-be careful of the bladder neck with this- it comes with a deflector that can rip tissue.

- A high-intensity (xenon) light source is used via a flexible fiberoptic cable to visualise the bladder and urethra (Akornor 2005).
- The telescope itself uses a rod lens system to transmit the images to the endoscopist- the air in-between the glass lenses acts as a refractory medium.
- The tip of the scope is angled from 0 (flat, for urethroscopy) to 120 degrees (retro view).
- The advantages of rigid cystoscopes include (Leyh and Hartung, 2005):
  - Large visual field
  - Wide working channel for guidewires, stents.
  - Irrigation channel with a large caliber, better flow and better vision
  - Attachments to the outer sheath for an Ellik evacuator- to allow easy access for clot evacuation
  - Easy handling and orientation during the procedure

9.1   Indications for Rigid Cystoscopy, Components, and Advantages

Cystoscopy allows for direct visualization of the urethra, urethral sphincter, prostate, bladder and ureteral orifices as part of diagnostic procedures (Figs. 9.2, 9.3, 9.4, 9.5, 9.6, 9.7, 9.8, 9.9, 9.10 and 9.11).

The diameter of rigid cystoscopes varies between 6 F and 27 F; the most commonly used in adults having a diameter ranging between 15 F and 25 F (Akornor et al., 2005). In UK practise this can vary between 17-22 fr.

The modern rigid cystoscope is composed of four pieces: light source, telescope, bridge, and sheath.

Sometimes the sheath will come separately- the Albarran sheath - be careful of the bladder neck with this- it comes with a deflector that can rip tissue.

A high-intensity (xenon) light source is used via a flexible fiberoptic cable to visualise the bladder and urethra (Akornor 2005).

The telescope itself uses a rod lens system to transmit the images to the endoscopist- the air in between the glass lenses acts as a refractory medium.

The tip of the scope is angled from 0 (flat, for urethroscopy) to 120 degrees (retro view).

The advantages of rigid cystoscopes include (Leyh and Harding, 2005):

•Large visual field

•Wide working channel for guidewires, stents.

•Irrigation channel with a large calibre, better flow and better vision

•attachments to the outer sheath for an Ellik evacuator- to allow easy access for clot evacuation

• Easy handling and orientation during the procedure

The external sheath allows easy insertion of the telescope and the irrigation fluid into the bladder.

When a therapeutic manoeuvre is expected, 24–27 F sheaths are preferred because they allow for an easy insertion of various instruments through the working channel

The sheath is fitted at its proximal end with two connectors (ports) for inflow and outflow.

9.2 Components of a Rigid Cystoscope

Fig. 9.2 Components of a Rigid Cystoscope-external sheath- 22 Fr

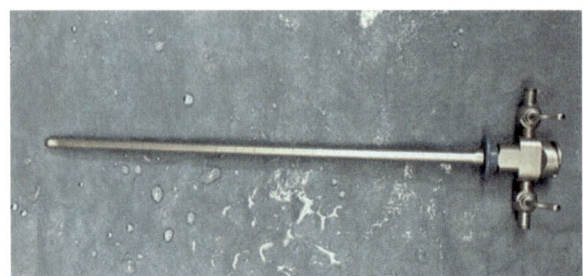

Fig. 9.3 Components of a Rigid Cystoscope- the 30 degree telescope

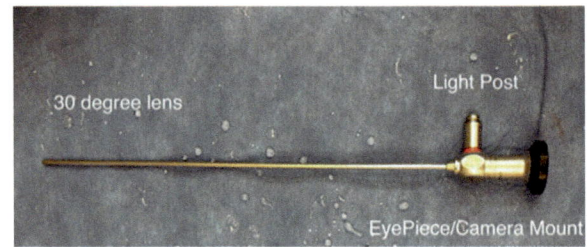

Fig. 9.4 Bridge, working channel and rod lens mount

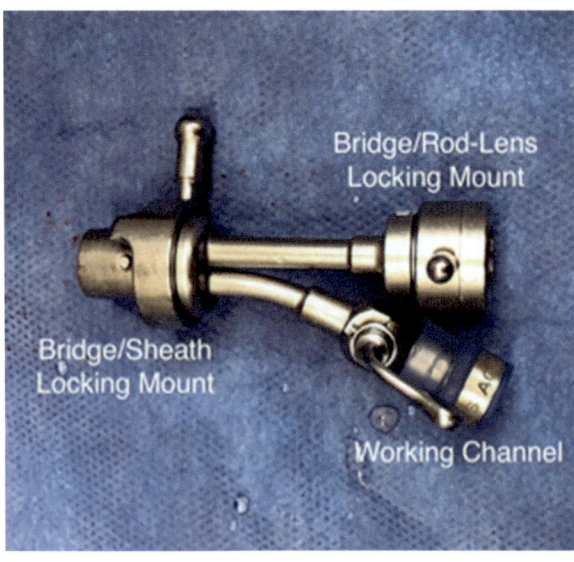

Fig. 9.5 The lens bridge
assembly

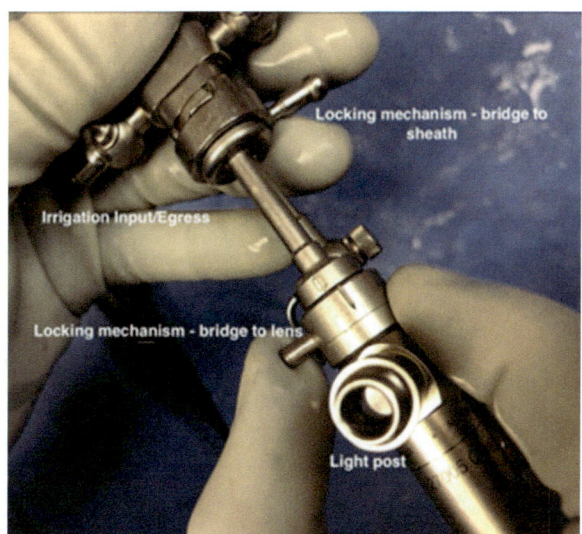

Fig. 9.6 The dual bridge

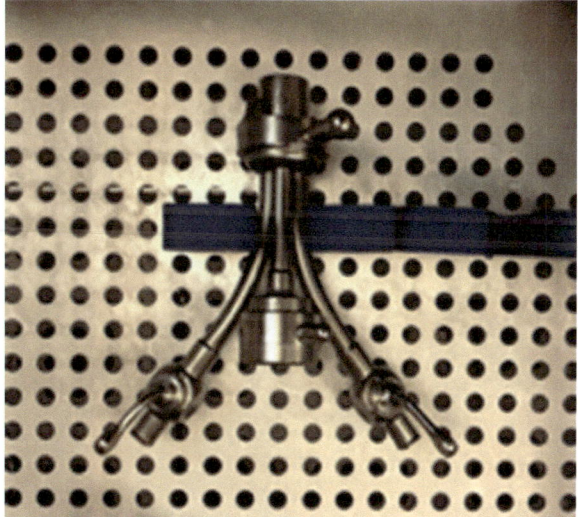

Fig. 9.7 Accessories for
the Rigid Cystoscope – the
light lead

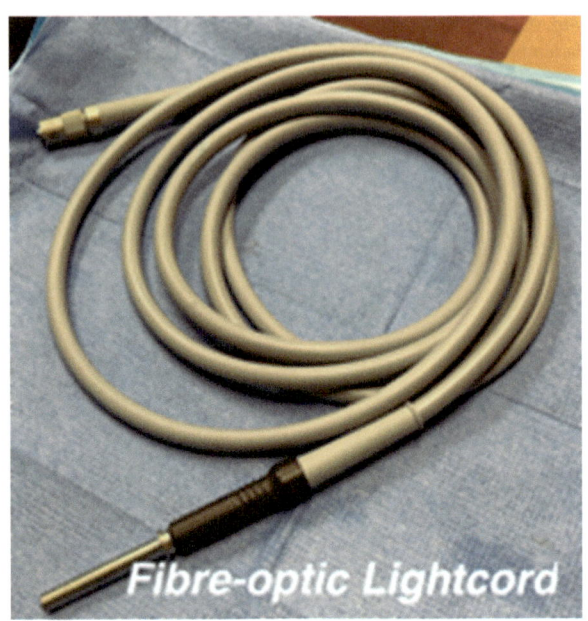

Fig. 9.8 The Camera

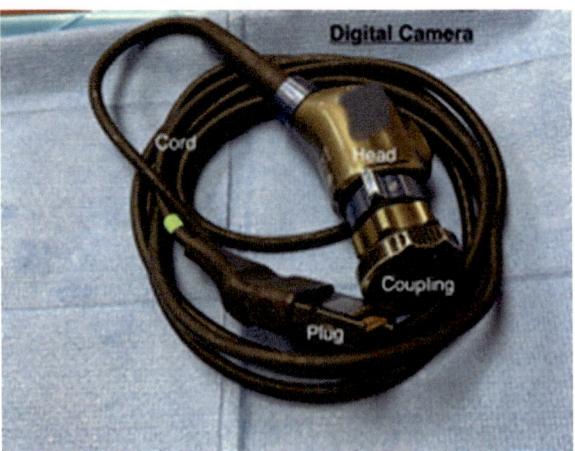

Fig. 9.9 The Stopcock -
irrigation connection

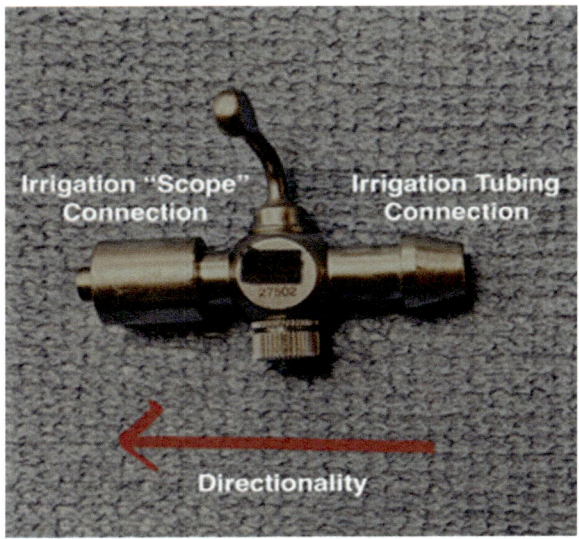

Fig. 9.10 The Rigid
Cystoscope Albarran
Bridge

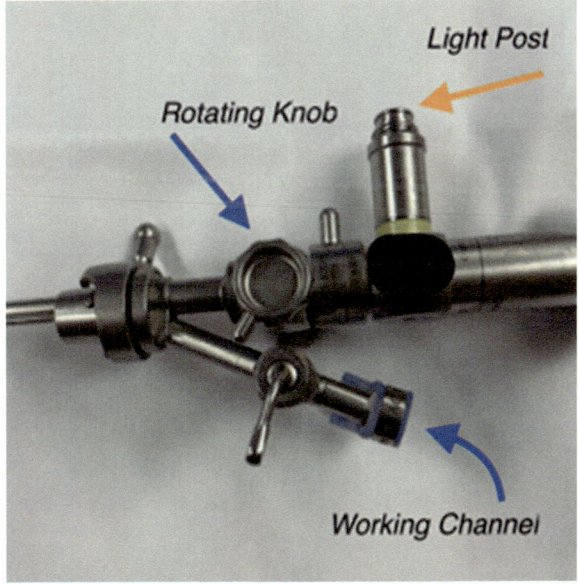

Fig. 9.11 Deflecting tip of the Albarran Bridge

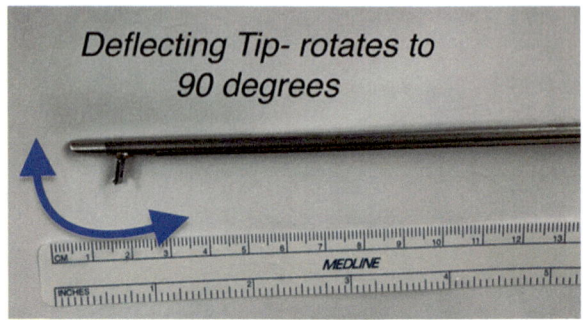

9.3   Instruments Used in the Rigid Cystoscopy, Components and Indications

Via the external sheath, several types of instruments may be used: biopsy forceps, guidewires, laser fibres, lithotripsy probes, injection needles, etc.

The Albarran sheath is an intermediate piece variant that is fitted with a distal deflecting system, which facilitates the handling of instruments that are introduced through the working channel in areas with difficult access.

The use of the Albarran sheath is avoided by some urologists because of the traumatic risk (mucosal lesions or perforations).

Degrees of lens 0° optical angle (forward view) are used particularly for urethroscopy

12–30° angles (forward and oblique view) are used especially for the examination of the base, posterior wall, and sidewalls of the bladder;

70° (side view) enable the examiner to view the anterolateral walls and the bladder dome.

120° angles (retrograde view) are used to inspect the anterior area of the bladder neck (Carter and Chan, 2007).

Uses
Bladder/ Prostate Assessment
Biopsy of bladder tumours
Lithoclast/ Laser to bladder stones
Clot evacuation
Removal of small stones
Difficult catheterisation
Botox injections
Placement of ureteric stents

References

Akornor JW, Segura JW, Nehra A. General and cystoscopic procedures. Urol Clin North Am. 2005 Aug;32(3):319–26.

Engelsgjerd JS, Deibert CM. Cystoscopy. StatPearls. 2019 Jan–2019 Jul 16. Treasure Island, FL: StatPearls Publishing

Leyh H, Hartung R. Internal Urethrotomy. Aktuelle Urol. 2005 Jun;36(3):271–8.

The Flexible Cystoscope

10

10.1 Medical Physics of the Flexible Cystoscope, Instruments and Advantages

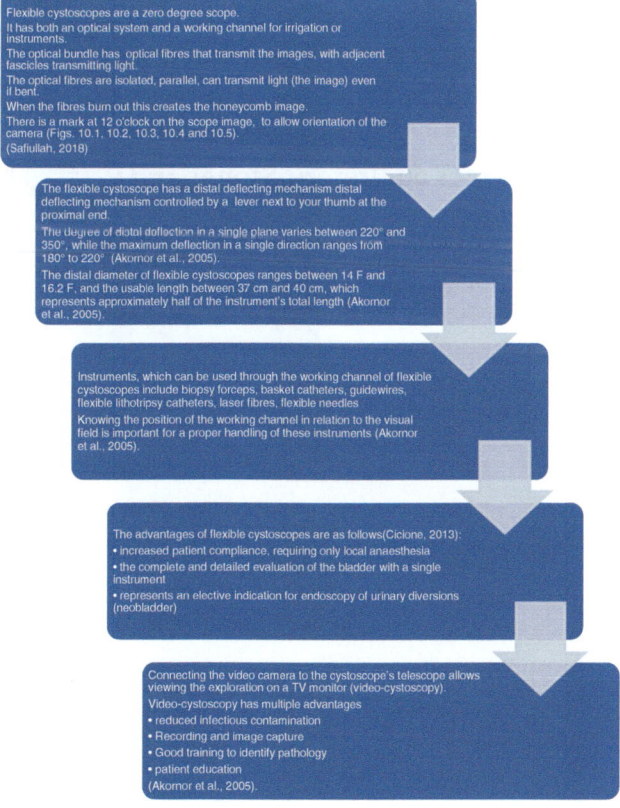

Flexible cystoscopes are a zero degree scope.
It has both an optical system and a working channel for irrigation or instruments.
The optical bundle has optical fibres that transmit the images, with adjacent fascicles transmitting light.
The optical fibres are isolated, parallel, can transmit light (the image) even if bent.
When the fibres burn out this creates the honeycomb image.
There is a mark at 12 o'clock on the scope image, to allow orientation of the camera (Figs. 10.1, 10.2, 10.3, 10.4 and 10.5).
(Safiullah, 2018)

The flexible cystoscope has a distal deflecting mechanism distal deflecting mechanism controlled by a lever next to your thumb at the proximal end.
The degree of distal deflection in a single plane varies between 220° and 350°, while the maximum deflection in a single direction ranges from 180° to 220° (Akornor et al., 2005).
The distal diameter of flexible cystoscopes ranges between 14 F and 16.2 F, and the usable length between 37 cm and 40 cm, which represents approximately half of the instrument's total length (Akornor et al., 2005).

Instruments, which can be used through the working channel of flexible cystoscopes include biopsy forceps, basket catheters, guidewires, flexible lithotripsy catheters, laser fibres, flexible needles
Knowing the position of the working channel in relation to the visual field is important for a proper handling of these instruments (Akornor et al., 2005).

The advantages of flexible cystoscopes are as follows(Cicione, 2013):
• increased patient compliance, requiring only local anaesthesia
• the complete and detailed evaluation of the bladder with a single instrument
• represents an elective indication for endoscopy of urinary diversions (neobladder)

Connecting the video camera to the cystoscope's telescope allows viewing the exploration on a TV monitor (video-cystoscopy).
Video-cystoscopy has multiple advantages
• reduced infectious contamination
• Recording and image capture
• Good training to identify pathology
• patient education
(Akornor et al., 2005).

S. S. Goonewardene et al., *Surgical Strategies in Endourology for Stone Disease*, https://doi.org/10.1007/978-3-030-82143-2_10

Fig. 10.1 A flexible
cystoscope

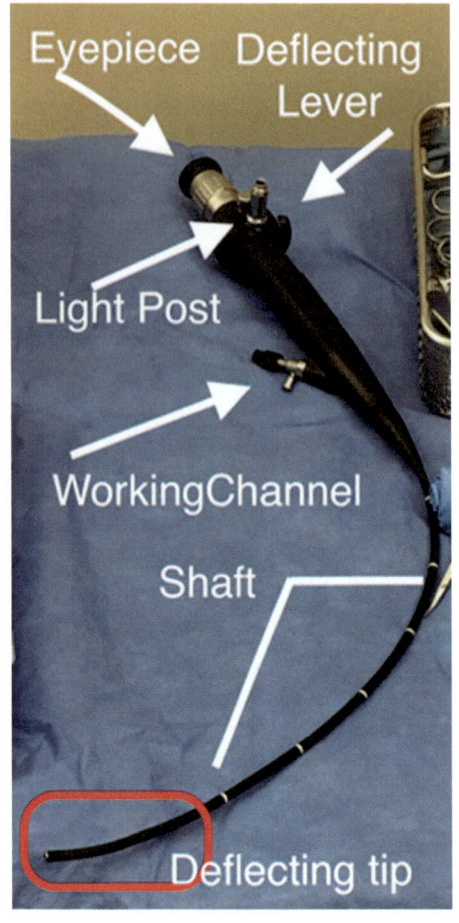

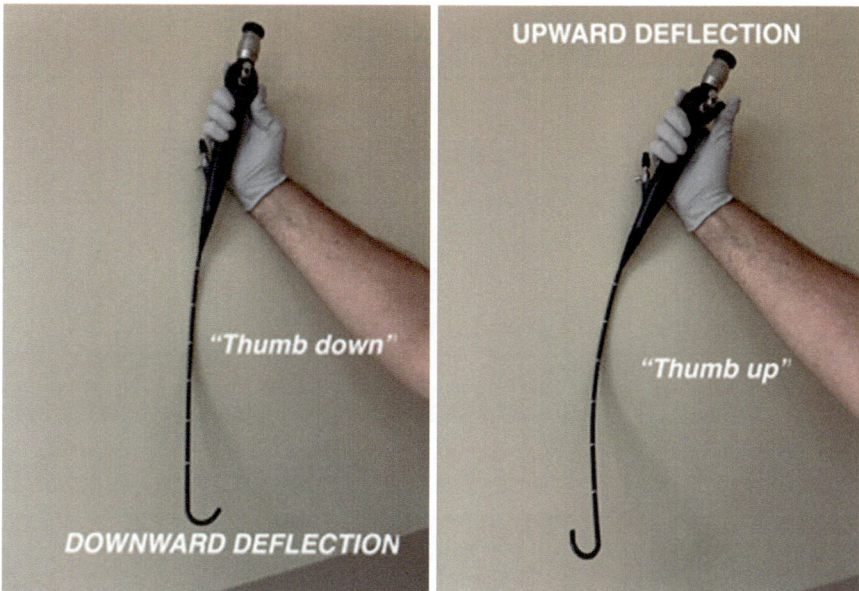

Fig. 10.2 Deflection in a flexible cystoscope

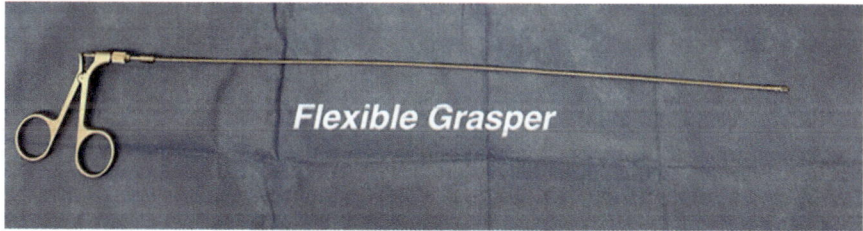

Fig. 10.3 Graspers used to remove stents during flexible cystoscopy

Fig. 10.4 Tip of flexible cystoscope

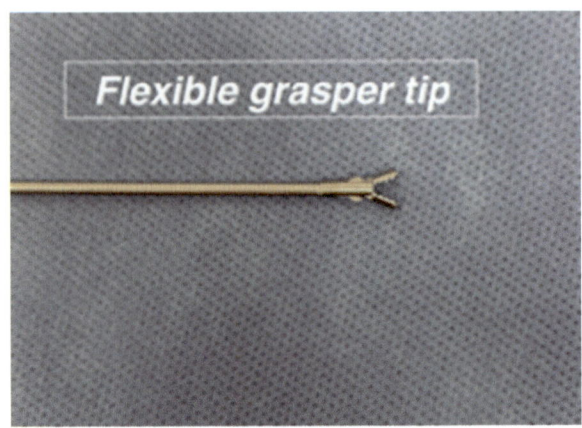

Fig. 10.5 The Working Channel in a Flexible Cystoscope

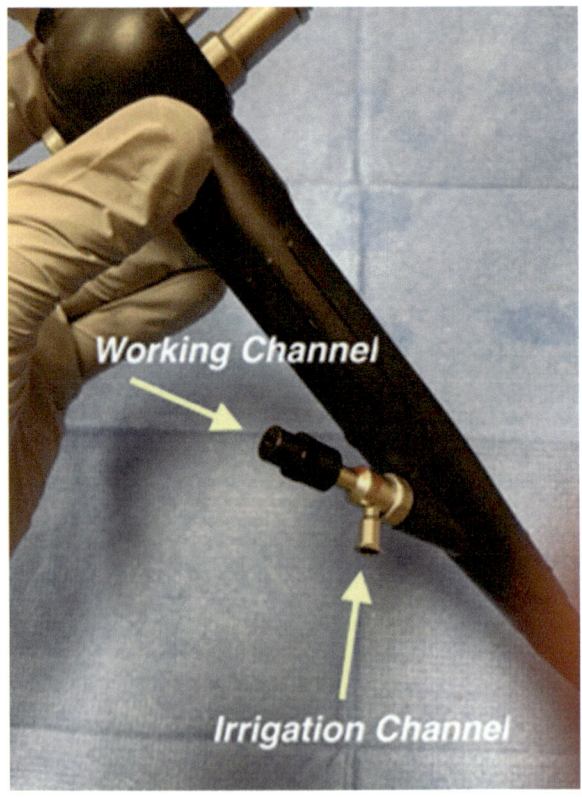

References

Akornor JW, Segura JW, Nehra A. General and cystoscopic procedures. Urol Clin North Am. 2005 Aug;32(3):319–26.

Cicione A, Cantiello F, Damiano R. Cystoscopy in non-muscle-invasive bladder cancer: when and how (rigid or flexible). Urologia. 2013;80(Suppl 21):11–5.

Safiullah S, Lama DJ, Patel R, Clayman RV. Procedural module: flexible cystoscopy. J Endourol. 2018 May;32(S1):S2–6.

The Rigid Ureteroscope

11.1 Medical Physics of the Rigid Ureteroscope

Rigid ureteroscopes are ideal for therapeutic procedures within the ureter and renal pelvis.

They have a cylindrical lens systems.

More modern endoscopes allows optic fibres that allow a significant reduction of dimensions,

However images are of a better quality using a cylindrical lens system.

After placement of the safety wire, the rigid ureteroscope would be passed, with a working wire as a proboscis.

The working wire would be passed to the renal pelvis.

Usually, a 9.5-Fr rigid ureteroscope is used first for optical dilation of the intramural and distal ureter (Akomor, 2005).

The scope would be passed between the two wires to the renal pelvis.

This manoeuvre allows for safe advancement of the ureteroscope in 95% of patients (Akomor, 2005).

The ureteroscope is normally a 5 degree scope, which may be short (33 cm) or long (45 cm).

The diameter varies between 13 F and 16 F.

Larger diameter working channels allow superior irrigation and visibility.

However, due to the diameter of over 10 F, the use of these instruments requires the dilatation of the ureteral orifice (Bagley, 2004), increasing the aggressiveness to the tissues.

The incidence of secondary ureteral stenoses after ureteroscopic manoeuvres is in direct correlation with the dimensions of the endoscope (Whitehurst, 2018).

S. S. Goonewardene et al., *Surgical Strategies in Endourology for Stone Disease*, https://doi.org/10.1007/978-3-030-82143-2_11

11.2   Rigid Ureteroscopy: Indications and Advantages

Huffman (1983) described a rigid ureteroscope with a cylindrical lens system, with an external diameter of 8.5 F and a working channel of 3.5 F.

Regarding the distal end's design, they are conical to allow ease of access to the intramural ureter.

The use of rigid optical systems determines distortions of image.

This can reduce the visual field by up to 50% (Miller et al., 1986).

It is important to check the scope, prior to insertion.

Rigid ureteroscopes that are disposable have now been produced as have sets with a removable telescope.

This means 0–70° optical systems can be used in the same sheath.

Integrated telescopes have a visual angle varying between 0° and 6.5°, allowing the ureteroscope's diameter to be reduced while maintaining a sufficient working channel (3.5–5 F).

Obtaining a visual angle of 6.5° allows for an easier orientation of the instruments when emerging from the working channel.

Uses of semi-rigid ureteroscopy

Management of ureteral strictures

Assessment of ureter- diagnostic ureteroscopy

Assessment of PUJO

Stone clearance

Ureteral biopsy, assessment of filling defects

Ureteroscopy may also contribute to the etiological diagnosis of obstructions at the ureteral or uretero-pelvic junction level.

11.3   Construct of a Rigid Ureteroscope

Figures 11.1 and 11.2 demonstrating construction of a rigid ureteroscope (Figs. 11.3, 11.4, 11.5, 11.6 and 11.7).

Fig. 11.1 The Storz Rigid Ureteroscopy with single working channel

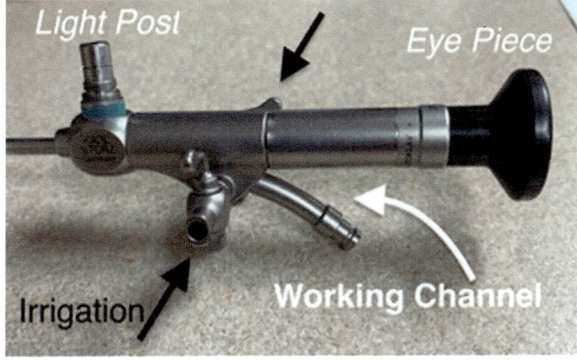

Fig. 11.2 The Storz full length rigid ureteroscopy

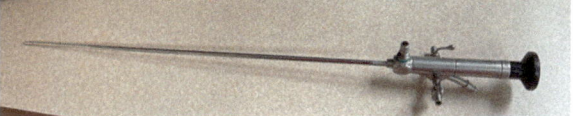

Fig. 11.3 Mid ureteric
stone, managed with a
rigid ureteroscope

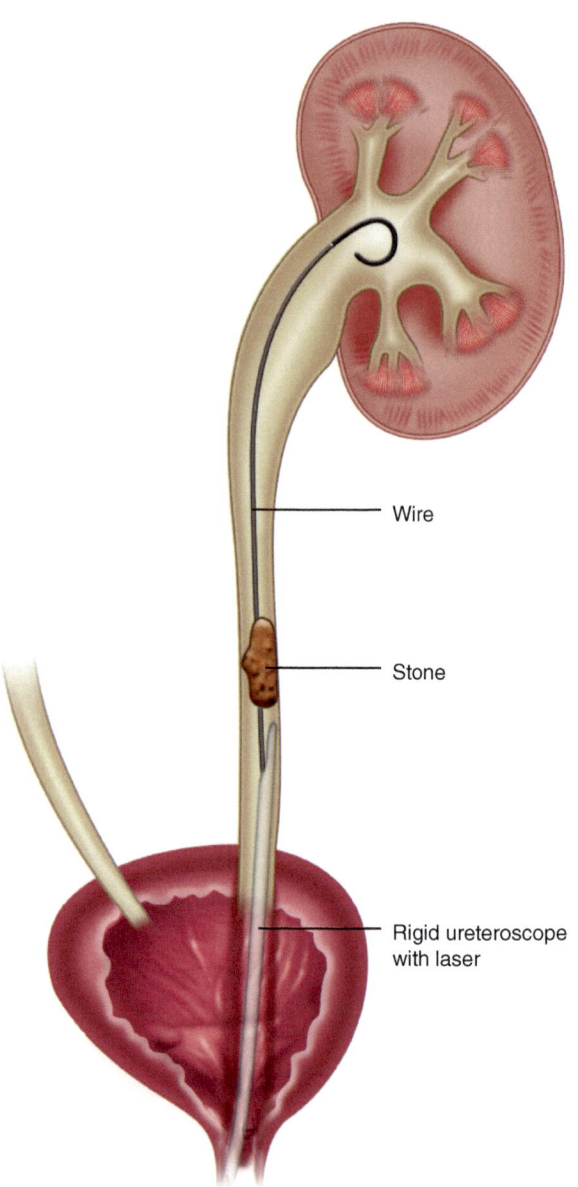

Wire

Stone

Rigid ureteroscope
with laser

Fig. 11.4 An Angle tipped
wire, to help negotiate
difficult wire insertion

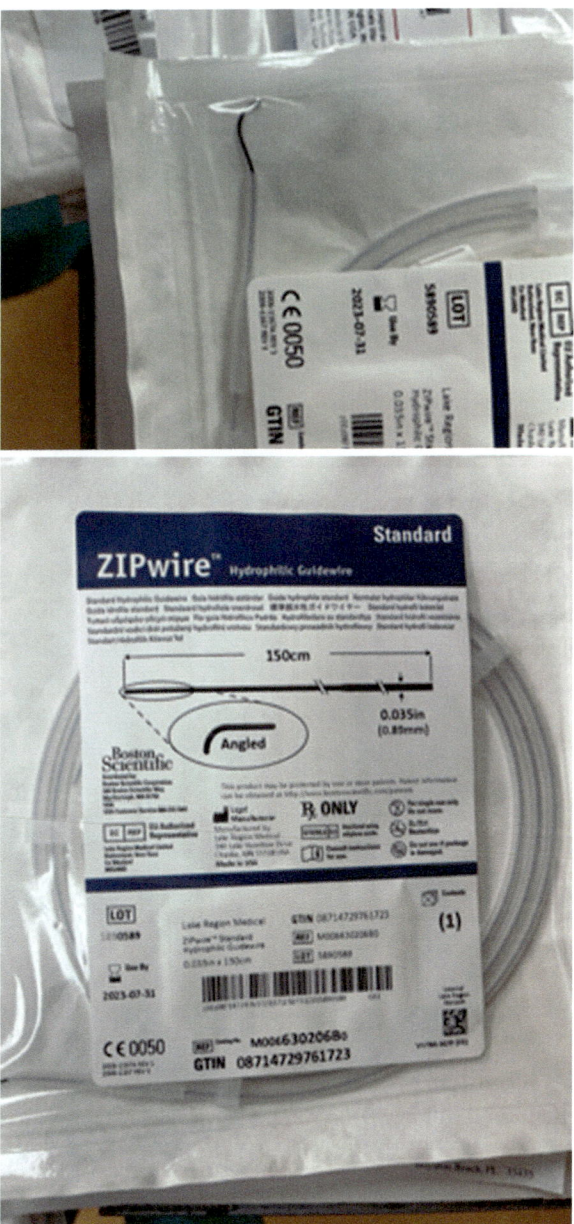

Fig. 11.5 The Olympus Rigid Ureterscope side view

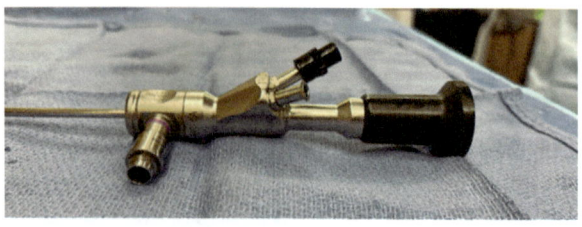

Fig. 11.6 The Olympus Rigid Ureteroscope—full length with. Dual channels

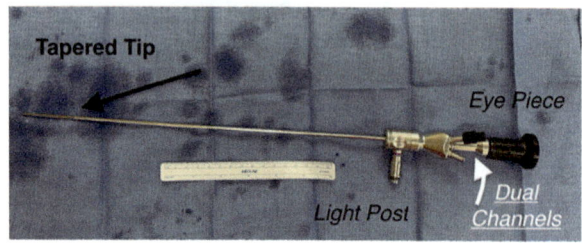

Fig. 11.7 The Olympus Rigid Ureteroscope dual channel, eye piece and light post

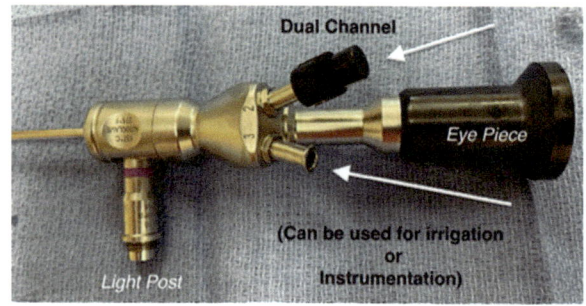

References

Akornor JW, Segura JW, Nehra A. General and cystoscopic procedures. Urol Clin North Am. 2005 Aug;32(3):319–26.

Bagley DH. Ureteroscopic surgery: changing times and perspectives. Urol Clin North Am. 2004 Feb;31(1):1–4.

Huffman JL, Bagley DH, Lyon ES. Extending cystoscopic techniques into the ureter and renal pelvis. Experience with ureteroscopy and pyeloscopy. JAMA. 1983 Oct 21;250(15):2002–5.

Miller RA, Ramsay JW, Crocker PR, Carter S, Eardley I, Whitfield HN, Wickham JE. Ureterorenal endoscopy: which instrument, what cost? Br J Urol. 1986 Dec;58(6):610–6.

Whitehurst LA, Somani BK. Semi-rigid ureteroscopy: indications, tips, and tricks. Urolithiasis. 2018 Feb;46(1):39–45.

Flexible Ureterorenoscopy

Management of urolithiasis

Urolithiasis is a significant worldwide source of morbidity, constituting a common urological disease that affects between 10 and 15% of the world population (Desai, 2017).

PCNL choice - stone factors (stone size, stone composition, and stone location), patient factors (habitus and renal anomalies), and failure of other treatment modalities (ESWL and flexible ureteroscopy) (Desai, 2017).

The accepted indications for PCNL are stones larger than 20 mm², staghorn and partial staghorn calculi, and stones in patients with chronic kidney disease (Desai, 2017).

Flexible ureteroscopy can be one of the options for lower pole stones between 1.5 and 2 cm in size (Desai, 2017). This option should be exercised in cases of difficult lower polar anatomy and ESWL-resistant stones. Flexible ureteroscopy can also be an option for stones located in the diverticular neck or a diverticulum (Desai, 2017).

ESWL is the treatment to be discussed as an option in all patient with renal stones (excluding lower polar stones) between size 10 and 20 mm. In addition, in lower polar stones of size between 10 and 20 mm if the anatomy is favourable, ESWL is the option. In proximal ureteral stones, ESWL should be considered as an option with flexible ureteroscopy (Desai, 2017).

Active monitoring has a limited role and can be employed in post-intervention (PCNL or ESWL) residual stones, in addition, asymptomatic patients with no evidence of infection and fragments less than 4 mm can be monitored actively (Desai, 2017).

S. S. Goonewardene et al., *Surgical Strategies in Endourology for Stone Disease*, https://doi.org/10.1007/978-3-030-82143-2_12

12.1   Flexible Uretero-Renoscope-Indication, Basic Principles, Ureteral Access Technique

Indication

- Lasering and extraction of renal stones
- As part of PCNL with a laser
- To biopsy and laser upper tract TCC
- (Figure 1-6- Flexible uretero-renoscope construct)

Basic principles

- Guidewire access
- Passage of ureterosocpe
- Accessing the stone
- Stone fragmentation / retrieval
- Establishing urinary drainage

Ureteral access

Initial retrograde pyelogram
- Pass 0.038 guidewire through ureteral stent, bypassing stone and coil within renal pelvis
- "Glidewire" used for tortuous ureter or impacted stone
- Advance catheter below stone to direct tip of wire
  Always replace slippery glidewire with standard Bentson or superstiff guidewire
- Place second (working) wire if therapeutic manoeuvres are anticipated (flexible URS)

The technique

- Initial retrograde pyelogram
- Passage of two 0.038" guidewires
       (safety & working)
- Dilation of intramural ureter (+/-)
- Passage of flexible ureteroscope over working wire
- Use of fluoroscopic monitoring to confirm position of wires and scope

12.2   Construct, Diameter, Working Channel Gauge and Deflection

Please see below Figs. 12.2, 12.3, 12.4, 12.5 and Table 12.1d for flexible ureteroscopes

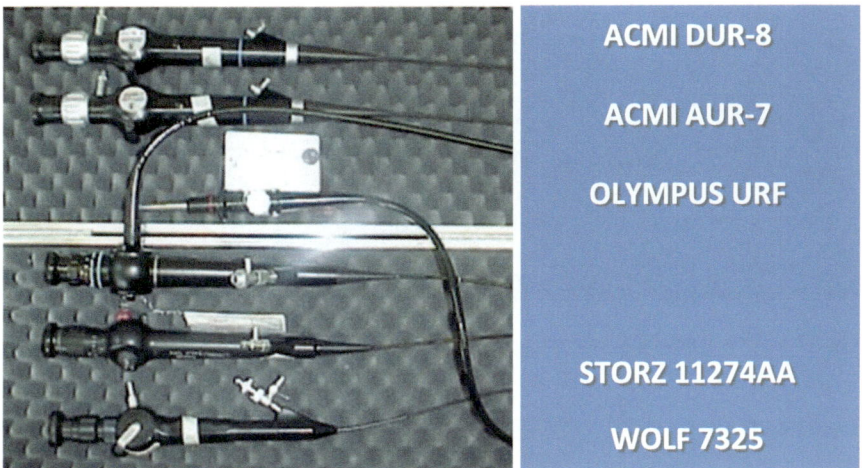

Fig. 12.1   Different flexible ureteroscopes

Fig. 12.2   The Flexible Ureteroscope

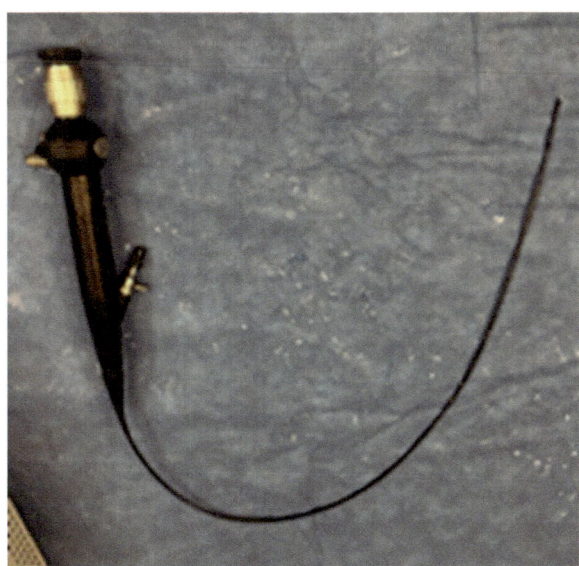

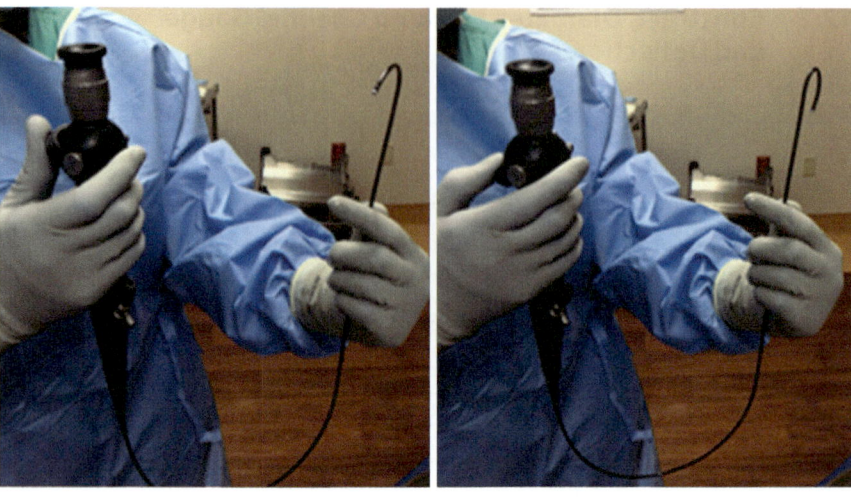

Fig. 12.3 How a flexible ureteroscope works Dual deflection 185 degrees down, 175 degrees up

Fig. 12.4 Thumb lever

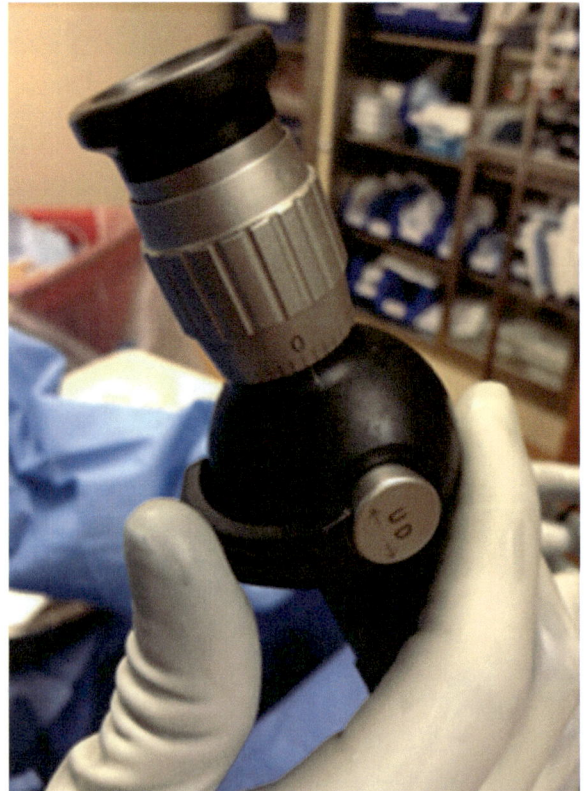

Fig. 12.5 The Pathfinder with Squeeze bulb, to maintain water pressure during ureteroscopy

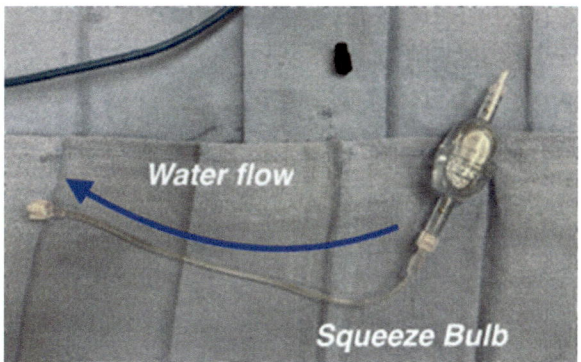

Table12.1 Flexible ureteroscopy comparison

Ureteroscope	Olympus-URF-P3	Storz 1124AA	Wolf 7325.172
Tip diameter	6.9F	7.5F	6.8F
Shaft diameter	8.4F	8.0F	7.5F
Working length	70 cm	70 cm	70 cm
Channel size	3.6F	3.6F	3.6F
Deflection up (degrees)	180	120	130
Deflection down (degrees)	100	170	160
Angle (degrees)	0	6	0

12.3   Light Transmission in the Flexible Uretero-Renoscope

The optical fibers of the three fascicles allow the accurate transmission of light and images despite bending

Of the three fascicles of optical fibres, two have a noncoherent structure (for light transmission) and one has a coherent structure (for image transmission) (Akomor, 2005).

The coherent bundle is formed from thousands of glass fibres so the image received at the distal end is transmitted identically to the proximal end.

This image has a lower resolution than a rigid nephroscopes, but has sufficient quality to allow their efficient use during endourological interventions.

In the recently developed digital flexible nephroscopes, this traditional optic system is replaced by a chip at the distal end. The image is transmitted digitally.

Thus, the inconveniences of the classic optical system are overcome (distorted image, low resolution, honeycomb aspect) while maintaining he endoscope's flexibility.

Enables you to get access with a second wire, by passing the catheter over the safety wire then passing a working wire (Figs. 12.6 and 12.7).

Fig. 12.6 The Dual
Lumen Catheter

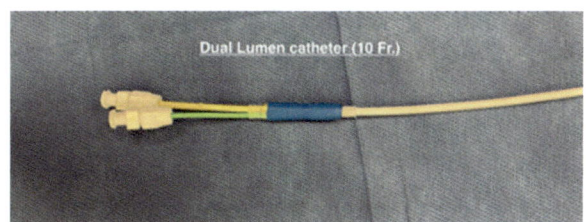

Fig. 12.7 Tip of the Dual
Lumen Catheter

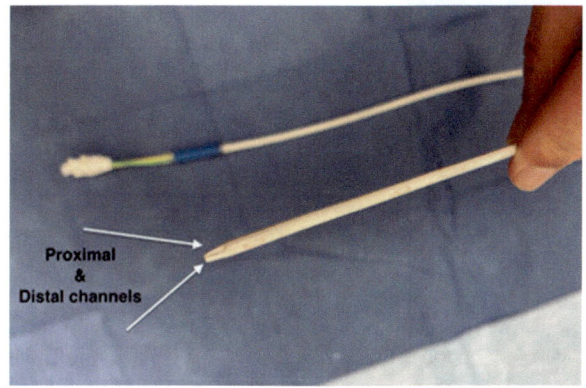

12.4   Access to the Renal Pelvis with the Flexible Ureteroscope

- Initial systems required placement of progressively larger dilating catheters followed by an 18 F access sheath
- First access systems reported a 19% perforation rate
- Trauma similar to graduated dilators
- Newer ureteral access sheaths availabl

DILATION OF The INTRAMURAL URETER

- When passing a flexible ureteroscope to the kidney, very often the intramural ureter must be dilated (Figs. 12.8, 12.9, 12.10, 12.11, 12.12, 12.13 and 12.14)
- This can be done using the following
- Metal cone-tipped bougies
- Graduated flexible dilators
- Flexible olive-tipped metal dilators
- Ureteral dilating balloon
- The dilating balloons, give a less traumatic dilation, with less bleeding or perforation risk.

FLUOROSCOPIC MONITORING

- Fluoroscopic monitoring is essential to confirm position of endoscope within the collecting system
- One can "outline" the collecting system on the fluoro monitor
- Reduces amount of infused contrast and xray usage

PASSAGE OF SCOPE

- Problem
  - Unable to pass the flexible ureteroscope up the ureter
- Solution
  - Dilate ureter more proximally
    Use ureteral access sheath
    Heavy-duty guidewire
    Place internal ureteral stent and bring patient back
            Come back in 7 - 14 days
- Anticipated (flexible URS)

The equipment

- Sensor wire 0.08 Fr- nitinol core over a hydrophilic coating
- Ureteric catheter- white (soft) or blue (stiffer)
- Contrast- Urograffin 150 or 300.
- Long rigid ureteroscope
- Flexible ureteroscope
- Access sheath

The strategy

- Rigid cystoscope in, with bridge
- Change to biopsy forceps
- Screen stent out, and pass sensor to renal pelvis
- Do a retrograde to see whether there are stones in the ureter
- Using the long rigid, clear the ureteric stones 1st.
- Alternatively, if ureter is clear of stones on screening, screen a flexible ureteroscope to the kidney
- Laser and clear lower pole stones
- Fragment and extract, start at 0.5/5 on laser settings
- 6x24 fr stent

The difficulties

- Flexion of the flexible cystoscopy to see the stone
- If a larger laser fibre than the 200 is used, it may result in poor flow and as a result, poor vision
- Stone must be repositioned in the midpole calyx, this is a better position for fragmentation
- Properly clearing stone, which may be in a dependant position- if the flexible cystoscope is maximally flexed, it is a difficult position to laser in.
- To get the best operative outcome, may the procedure straightforward.

The outcome

- Stones fully cleared from kidney.
- Chase stone type.
- Stent register- tract stent and ensure it is removed.
- Dietary advice including BAUS information leaflet.
- TFTs, Calcium, Urate .

Fig. 12.8 Passage of
flexible ureteroscope over
a guidewire, with a
safety wire

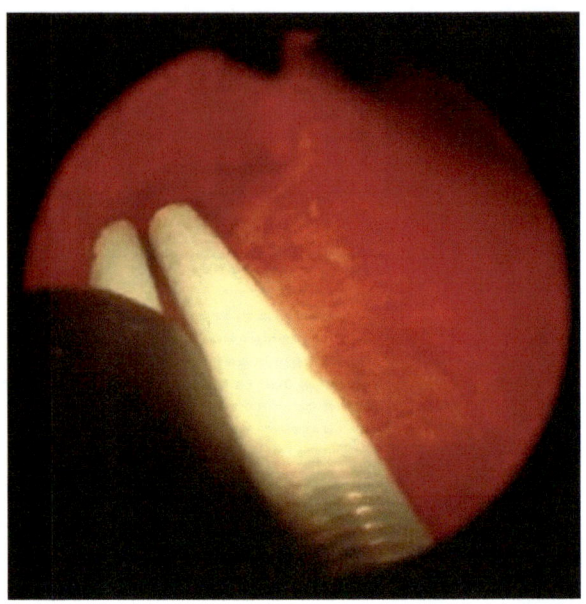

Fig. 12.9 Retrograde
pyelogram demonstrating
collecting system

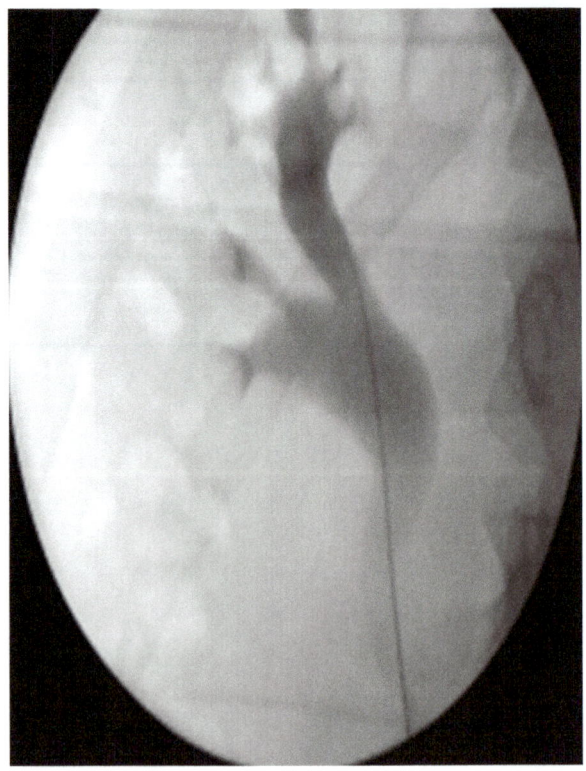

Fig. 12.10 Scope being advanced to the kidney with retrograde

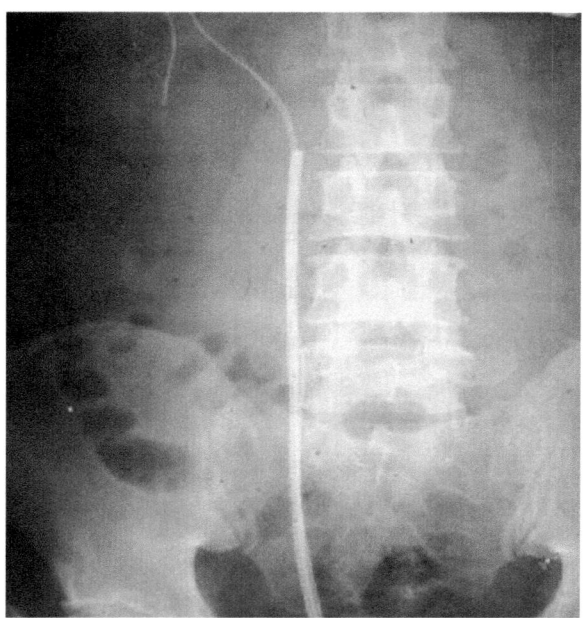

Fig. 12.11 Flexible ureteroscope in kidney

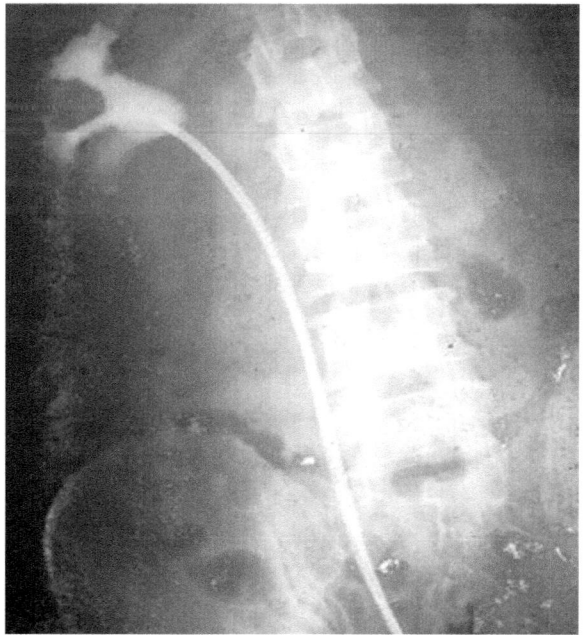

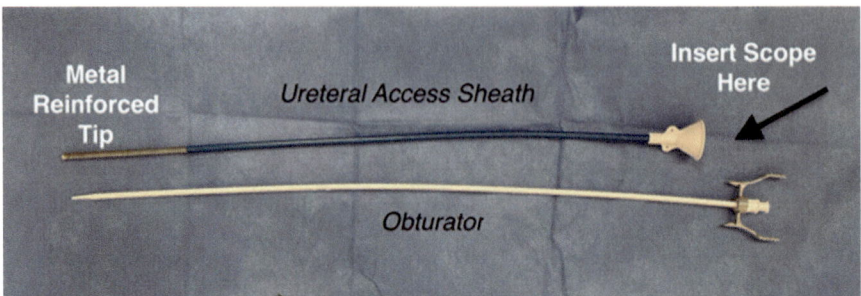

Fig. 12.12 Ureteral access sheath- with trochar in place

Fig. 12.13 Fluoroscopy
demonstrating sheath
above iliac vessels

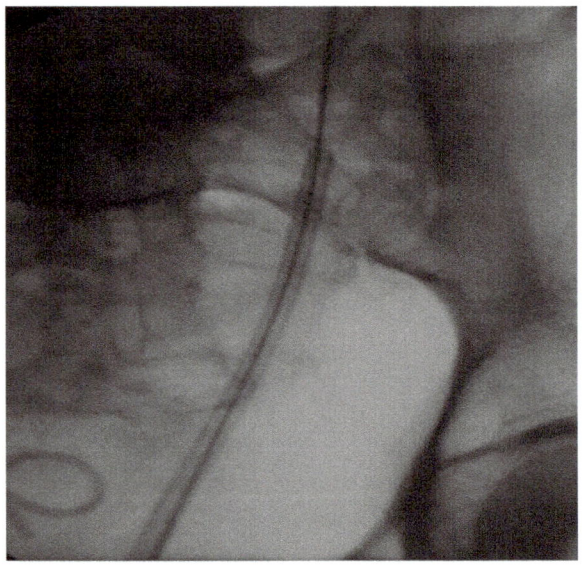

Fig. 12.14 Flexible
ureteroscopy through
access sheath

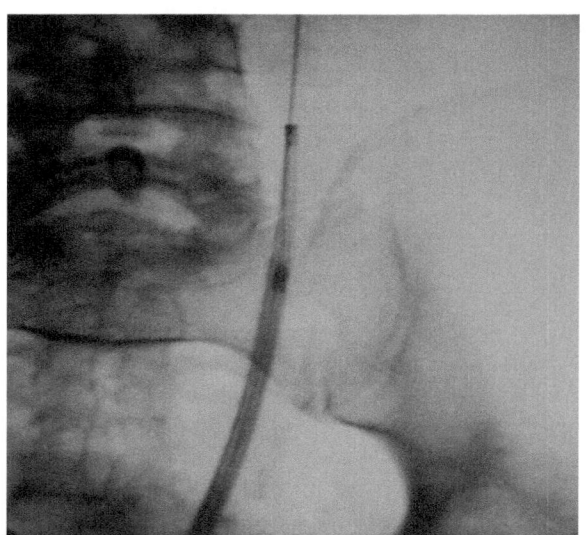

Surgical Strategy for Lower Pole Stones

13

13.1 Management Options in Lower Pole Renal Stones

Kidney stone disease is increasing worldwide with its most common location being in the lower pole (Moore, 2016).

For asymptomatic small lower pole stones, SWL and F-URS are established treatment modalities. However, conservative management is also an option (Sener, 2015).

Ureteroscopy has a key role in management of lower pole stones.

NICE Guidelines 2019 for Renal stones
Offer SWL
Consider URS:
if there are contraindications for SWL **or**
if a previous course of SWL has failed **or**
because of anatomical reasons, SWL is not indicated
Consider PCNL if SWL and URS have failed to treat the current stone or they are not an option

- Consider URS or SWL
- Consider PCNL if:
- URS or SWL have failed **or**
- for anatomical reasons, PCNL is the more favourable option

© The Author(s), under exclusive license to Springer Nature Switzerland AG 2021
S. S. Goonewardene et al., *Surgical Strategies in Endourology for Stone Disease*,
https://doi.org/10.1007/978-3-030-82143-2_13

13.2   Micro PCNL vs. Retrograde Renal Surgery for Lower Pole Stones

Kandemir reviewed micropercutaneous nephrolithotomy (microperc) and retrograde intrarenal surgery (RIRS) for the management of lower pole kidney stones up to 15 mm (Kandemir, 2017). The mean stone size was 10.6 (5-15) and 11.5 (7-15) mm for Microperc and RIRS groups, respectively (P = 0.213) (Kandemir, 2017). In the Microperc group, the scopy time was 158.5 s, while in the RIRS group, the scopy time was 26.6 s (P = 0.001) (Kandemir, 2017). The hospitalization period in the Microperc group was 542 h, while it was 19 h in the RIRS group (P = 0.001) (Kandemir, 2017).

No statistical differences were observed during the operating time, pre-operative-post-operative haemoglobin (Hb), serum creatinine, and estimated glomerular filtration speed (e-GFR) values and stone-free rates (Kandemir, 2017). No intraoperative complications were observed in either of the groups, while post-operative complications were observed in six patients in Microperc Group and five patients belonging to the RIRS Group (P = 0.922) (Kandemir, 2017).

Both Microperc and RIRS are safe and effective alternatives, and have similar stone clearance and complication rates for the management of lower pole kidney stones up to 15 mm in diameter (Kandemir, 2017).

13.3   Case 1

The case
- 36 year old male
- Admitted with renal colic
- Stent inserted 28/7/18
- No op note/ stent size on system   .

The condition
- 5 mm right lower pole stone
- 5 mm Proximal ureteric stone
- 3 mm proximal ureteric stone

Pre-operative imaging
- CT KUB
- Prior pyelogram (Figs. 13.1 and 13.2 for preoperative imaging and how to approach a lower pole stone)

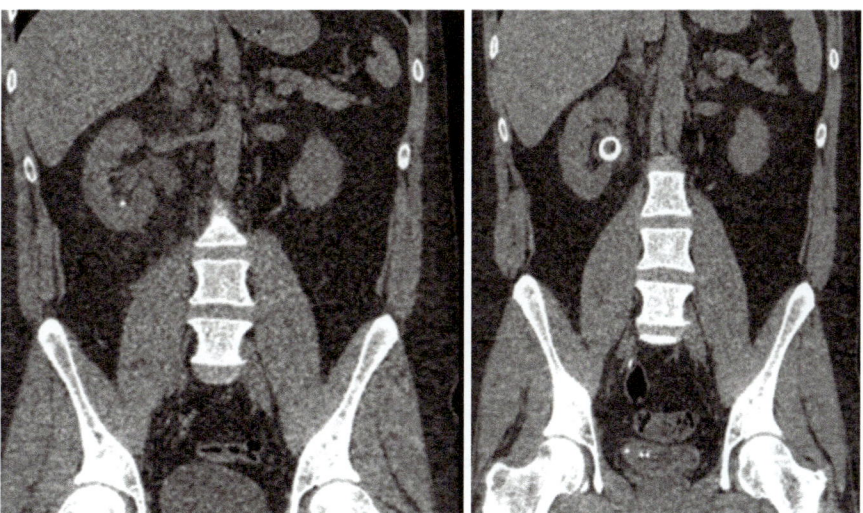

Fig. 13.1   CT KUB demonstrating lower pole stone, with ureteric stent

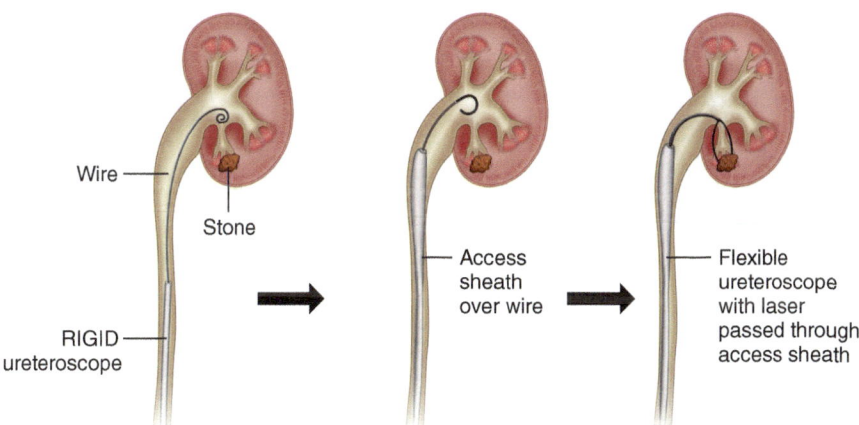

Fig. 13.2   How to approach a lower pole stone

13.4   Case 2

The case
- 70 year old male
- No information in records
- No letters from urology
- Cardiopath

The condition
- Right 6mm ureteric stone
- Emergency Stent
- Size unknown- op note not on system

Pre-operative imaging
- CT KUB
- Figures 13.3 and 13.4 for preoperative imaging

Pre-op surgical strategy
- Rigid cystoscope in, with bridge (Figures 3-10 for equipment)
- Pass sensor to renal pelvis, switch to biopsy forceps, screen stent out
- Do a retrograde to see whether there are stones in the ureter
- Using the long rigid with a 2nd sensor wire, make sure the ureter is clear 1st.
- Screen up a 45 10/12fr access sheath and railroad up the flexible ureterorenoscope
- Fragment and extract, start at 0.5/5 on laser settings
- Consider using engage to extract stones from calyces. 7 fr Multi-length stent

The equipment

- Sensor wire 0.08 Fr- nitinol core over a hydrophilic coating
- Ureteric catheter- white (soft) or blue (stiffer)
- Contrast- Urograffin 150 or 300.
- Long rigid ureteroscope
- Flexible ureteroscope
- Access sheath

The strategy

- Rigid cystoscope in, with bridge
- Do a retrograde to see whether there are stones in the ureter
- Sensor to right renal pelvis
- Using the long rigid, clear the ureteric stones 1st.
- Access sheath-10/12
- Laser and clear lower pole stones by moving to midpole
- Fragment and extract, start at 0.4/10 on laser settings
- 6x26 fr stent

The difficulties

- Flexion of the flexible cystoscopy to see the stone
- Stone must be repositioned in the midpole calyx, this is a better position for fragmention
- Properly clearing stone, which may be in a dependant position
- Do not laser in the lower pole
- If stone 1 cm or less for urs, if > 1cm- PCNL.
- URS strategy- wire to RP. Ureteric Cath and retrograde.
- Fragment and extract. Stent. Be prepared for 2nd procedure.

The outcome

- Stones fully cleared from kidney.
- Chase stone type.
- Stent register- tract stent and ensure it is removed.
- Dietary advice including BAUS information leaflet.
- TFTs, Calcium, Urate.

Fig. 13.3 CT
Demonstrating 6 Mm right
lower pole stone

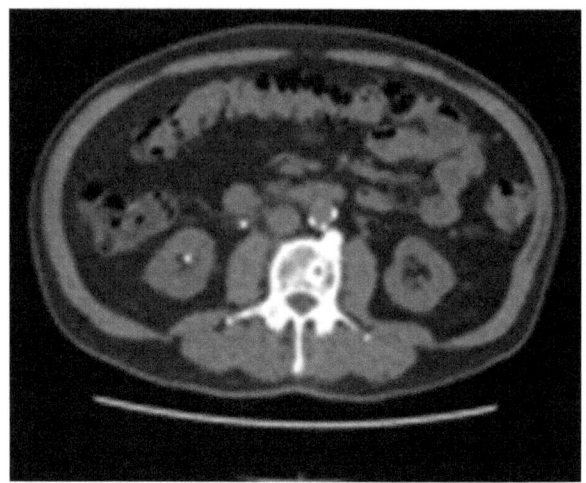

Fig. 13.4 CT
Demonstrating 6 Mm right
lower pole stone

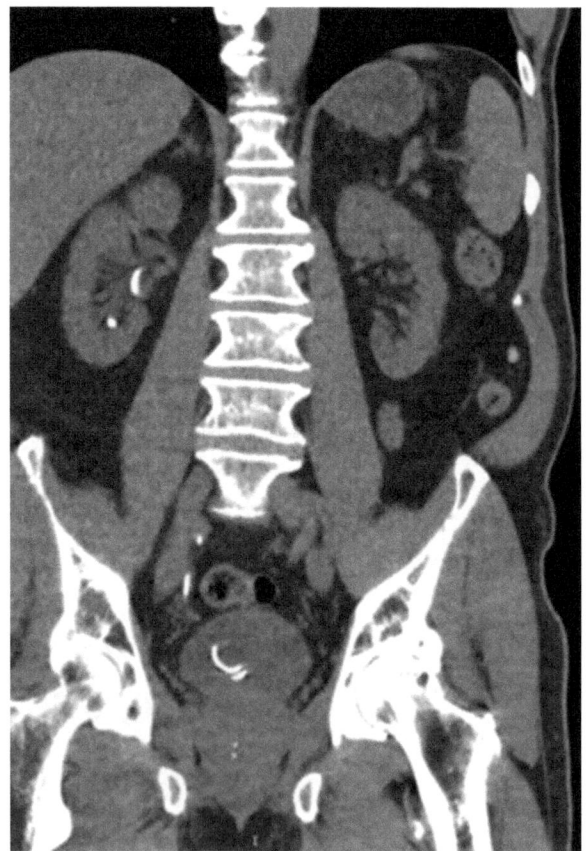

Plesae see (Figs. 13.5, 13.6, 13.7, 13.8, 13.9, 13.10, 13.11) and Table 13.1

Fig. 13.5 Guidewire
placement at end of
operation prior to stenting

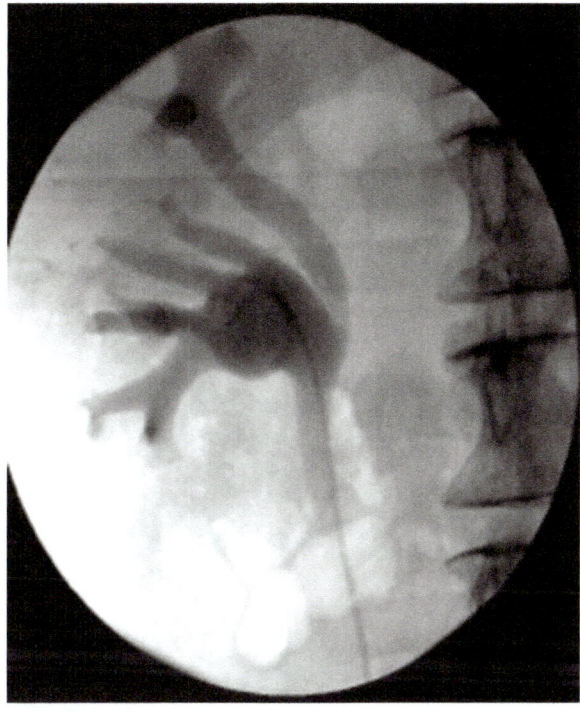

Fig. 13.6 A zero tip
basket—Open

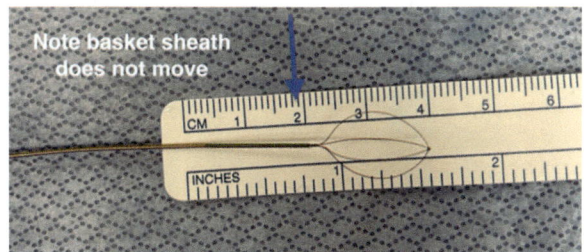

Fig. 13.7 A zero tip
Basket—Closed

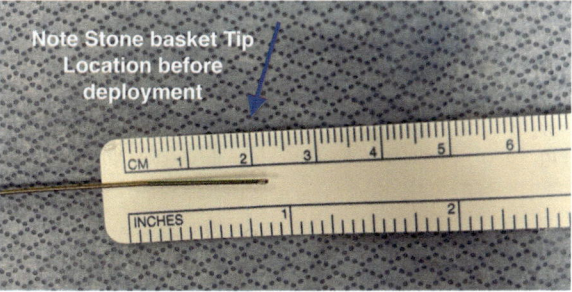

Fig. 13.8 The basket
handle

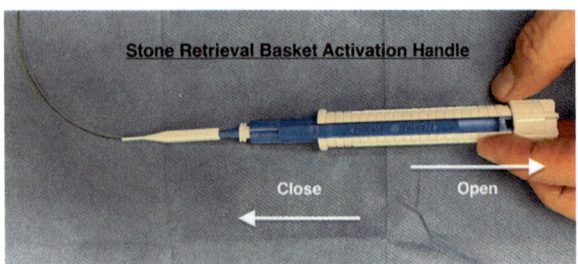

Fig. 13.9 The flexible
Ureterorenoscope

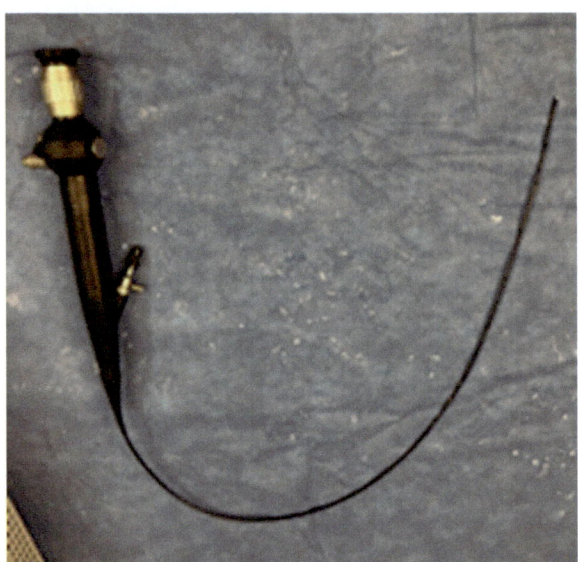

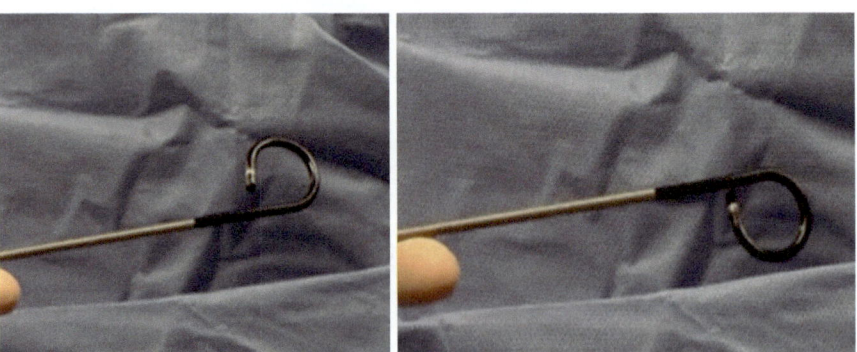

Fig. 13.10 Maximal deflection with a disposable Ureterorenoscope

Fig. 13.11 The Pathfinder- for improved vision during flexible Ureterorenoscopy

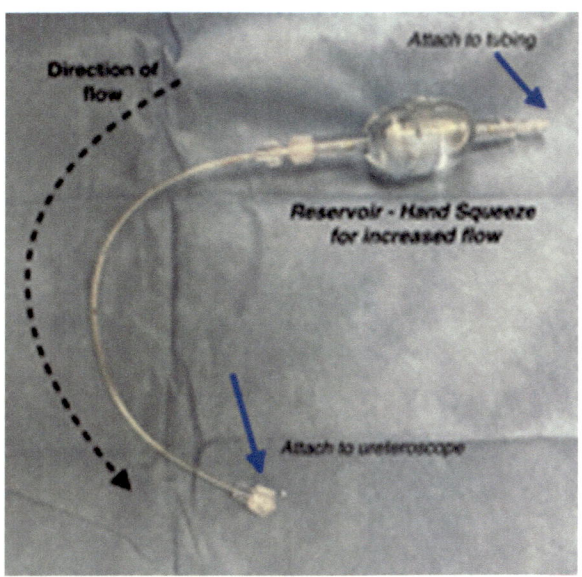

Table 13.1 Impact of Fibre diameter on scope deflection

Fibre diameter (Micrometers)	200	365
Karl Storz	7%	18%
Circon AUR-7	16%	37%

Kuo et al. (1998)

13.5   **Case 3** (Figs. 13.12, 13.13, 13.14 and Table 13.2)

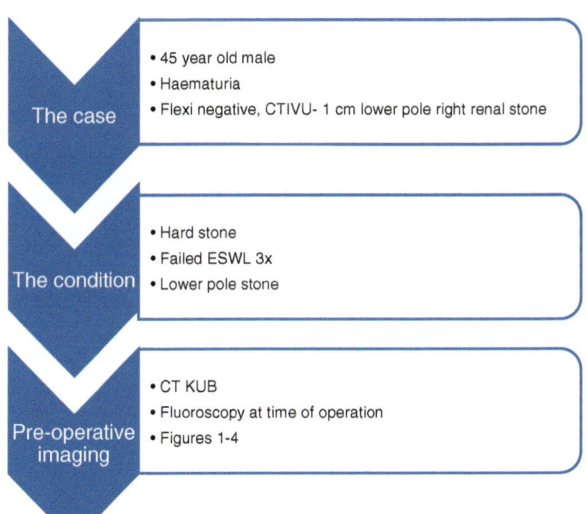

The case
- 45 year old male
- Haematuria
- Flexi negative, CTIVU- 1 cm lower pole right renal stone

The condition
- Hard stone
- Failed ESWL 3x
- Lower pole stone

Pre-operative imaging
- CT KUB
- Fluoroscopy at time of operation
- Figures 1-4

The equipment

- Sensor wire 0.08 Fr- nitinol core over a hydrophilic coating
- Ureteric catheter- white (soft) or blue (stiffer)
- Contrast- Urograffin 150 or 300.
- Long rigid ureteroscope
- FLexible ureteroscope
- Access sheath 45 long, 10/12 fr
- Xray, laser

The strategy

- Rigid cystoscope in, with bridge
- Pass sensor to renal pelvis., alongside stent, then screen stent out
- Do a retrograde to see whether there are stones in the ureter
- Using the long rigid, do a diagnostic ureteroscopy to view all areas of the ureter
- If ureter clear pass access sheath, railroad flexi and fragment stone
- If in good position you may be able to laser with long rigid alone, but always have access sheath and flexible ureteroscopy on standby.
- Do not force the access sheath as the ureter can be tight
- 6x24 fr stent (female patient, shorter stent)

The difficulties

- Favorable anatomy for lower pole stones- Angle > 70°·i width ≥ 5 mm, length ≤ 3 cm
- Unfavourable anatomy- Unfavorable anatomy Angle < 70, width < 5 mm, length > 3 cm
- Sometimes, stones are hiding in calyceal diverticula- if this is the case, the neck of the diverticula needs to be lasered open to access the stone.
- Other alternate methods include partial renorrhaphy to access to the stone.
- Get the stone into a better position- it is easier to laser in the midpole region, not a full flexion, when the stone is in the lower pole.

The outcome

- The lower pole stone was successfully cleared
- The patient was discharged home the same day
- BAUS dietary advice was given, especially to drink > 2.5L of water per day.
- As an initial stone former, bloods were sent for TFTs, PTH, calcium and urate

Fig. 13.12 CT KUB demonstrating right lower pole stone

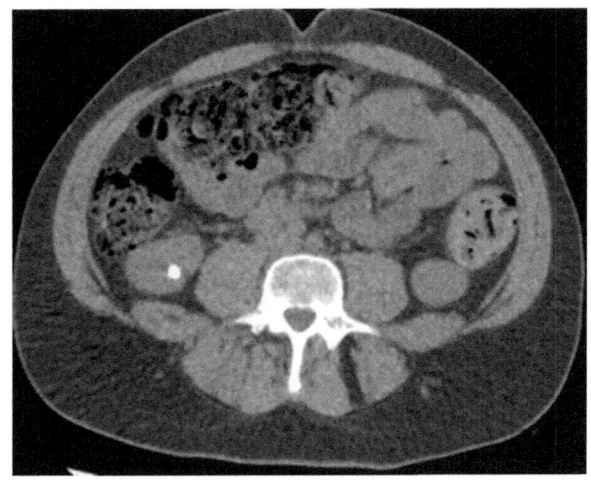

Fig. 13.13 CT KUB demonstrating right lower pole stone

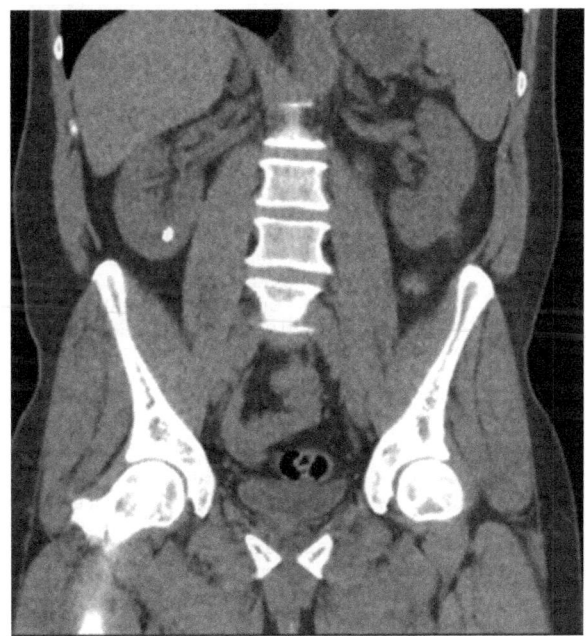

Fig. 13.14 Stone
demonstrated on
Fluoroscopy

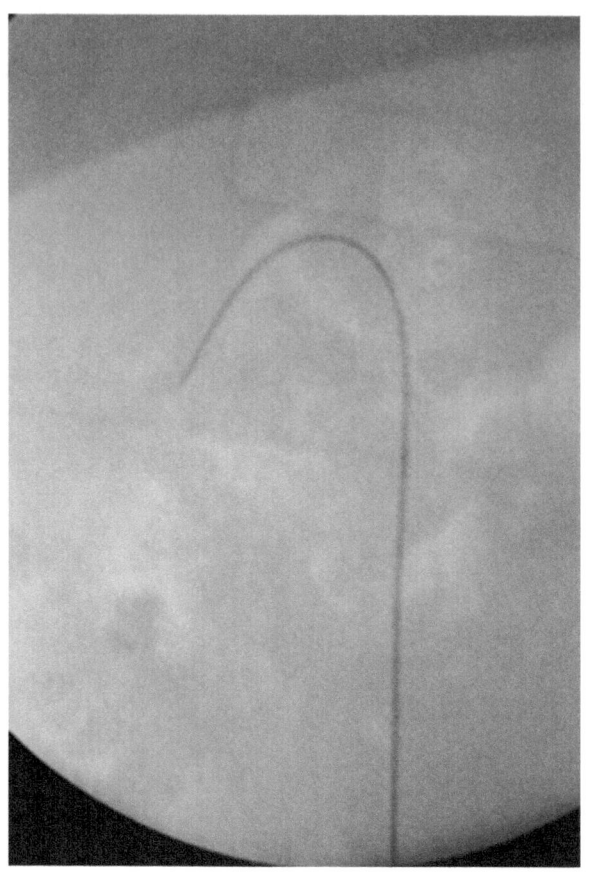

Table 13.2 Outcomes from ureteroscopy- insitu vs. displacement

	In-situ	Displacement
Stone diameter (mm)	8.0	10.3[a]
Operative time	64	80[a]
Stone free - total	71%	94%
<1 cm	77%	89%
>1 cm	29%	100%[a]

[a]P < 0.05 Hollenbeck et al. (2002)

13.6   Patient Information and Consent: What to Tell the Patient

Why is this procedure being done?

- This procedure is being done to remove stones from the lower pole of the kidney using a camera through the bladder
- Stones are broken up using a laser
- This procedure is done with cameras to avoid more major operations such as open surgery for stone removal
- A stent will be required at the end of the procedure, which may be removed in a few days (stent on strings) or a couple of weeks using a camera

What are the alternatives

- Conservative management
- ESWL- shock wave therapy to the stone to try and break it up- may require 2 sessions, f this fails, usually surgery is required
- PCNL- using a camera through the back into the kidney, very large stones can be extracted
- Robotic or laparoscopic stone surgery- not commonly done for stones
- Open stone surgery- not commonly done for stones

What the procedure entails

- A general anaesthetic is used
- Antibiotics are given pre-procedure
- A camera is inserted and contrast studies are done
- A camera and laser will be passed to the kidney
- The stone will be broken to fragments or removed or dusted
- A stent will be passed up to the kidney that will be removed at a later date

The outcome

- Infection, sepsis, HDU/ ITU stay
- Bleeding
- Recurrence
- Remnant stone requiring further treatment
- Failure to reach stone requiring stenting and a 2nd look procedure or nephrostomy
- Trauma to the ureter- abrasion, stricture, mucosal damage, ureteric reconstruction
- Anaesthetic risks - MI, CVA, PE, DVT, Chest infection

13.7   Asymptomatic Small Renal Stones

Prevalence of asymptomatic small renal stones- 3-5% (PAK, 1998)
US based survey- 5,047 patients, CT colonoscopy screening
3-5 mm mean stone size of 3mm.
2 stones per patient
21% having one symptomatic sdfsdfdsfstone episode in 10 years
(Boyce t al. 2010)

The *natural history* of small, non-obstructing asymptomatic calculi is not well defined, and the risk of progression is unclear.

There is still no consensus on the follow-up duration, timing and type of intervention.

Treatment options are chemolysis or active stone removal.

107, over 31 months- Symptomatic event in only 32% (Glowaki, 2002)

68% remained symptom free with numbers of stones and past history of stones being predictors of observation failure (Glowaki, 2002)

If patients were symptomatic – 47% passed their stone spontaneously, 26.5% required surgical intervention, 26.5% had ESWL (Glowaki, 2002)

300 patients, mean follow-up of 38 months (Burger, 2004)

77% progressed re stone size, number, and symptoms

26% required an intervention

Stones larger than 4mm or lower pole stones- likely to increase in size, develop symptoms or required intervention

References

Boyce CJ, Pickhardt PJ, Lawrence EM, Kim DH, Bruce RJ. Prevalence of urolithiasis in asymptomatic adults: objective determination using low dose noncontrast computerized tomography. J Urol. 2010;183(3):1017–21.

Byrne RR, Auge BK, Kourambas J, Munver R, Delvecchio F, Preminger GM. Routine ureteral stenting is not necessary after Ureteroscopy and Ureteropyeloscopy: a randomized trial. J Endourol. 2002;16(1):9–13.

Glowacki LS, Beecroft ML, Cook RJ, Pahl D, Churchill DN. The natural history of asymptomatic urolithiasis. J Urol. 2002;147(2):319–2.

Hollenbeck BK, Schuster TG, Faerber GJ, Wolf JS Jr. Comparison of outcomes of Ureteroscopy for ureteral calculi located above and below the pelvic brim. Urology. 2002;58(3):351–6.

Kandemir A, Guven S, Balasar M, Sonmez MG, Taskapu H, Gurbuz R. A prospective randomized comparison of micropercutaneous Nephrolithotomy (microperc) and retrograde intrarenal surgery (RIRS) for the management of lower pole kidney stones. World J Urol. 2017;35(11):1771–6.

Kuo RL, Aslan P, Fitzgerald KB, Preminger GM. Use of Ureteroscopy and holmium:YAG laser in patients with bleeding diatheses. Clinical Trial Urology. 1998;52(4):609–13.

Moore SL, Bres-Niewada E, Cook P, Wells H, Somani BK. Optimal management of lower pole stones: the direction of future travel. Cent European J Urol. 2016;69(3):274–9.

NICE Guideline. Renal and ureteric stones: assessment and management: NICE (2019) Renal and ureteric stones: assessment and management. BJU Int. Feb 2019;123(2):220–32.

Pak CY. Kidney stones. Lancet. 1998;351(9118):1797–801.

Sener NC, Bas O, Sener E, Zengin K, Ozturk U, Altunkol A, Evliyaoglu Y. Asymptomatic lower pole small renal stones: shock wave lithotripsy, flexible ureteroscopy, or observation? A prospective randomized trial. Urology. 2015 Jan;85(1):33–7.

Surgical Strategy for Renal Stones with Distal Ureteric Calculus

14.1   NICE Guidelines on Ureteric Stones and Dietary Advice

NICE Guidelines 2019, for large 10-20mm ureteric stones

Offer URS
Consider SWL if local facilities allow stone clearance within 4 weeks
Consider PCNL for impacted proximal stones when URS has failed

In children or young adults consider URS or SWL

NICE Guidelines 2019 Dietary advice
Discuss diet and fluid intake- drink 2.5 to 3 litres of water
per day, and children and young people (depending on their
age) 1 to 2 litres
Consider adding fresh lemon juice to drinking water
Avoid carbonated drinks

•Adults daily salt intake up to 6 g, and children and young
people (depending on their age) from 2 to 6 g
•Maintain a normal calcium intake of 700 to 1,200 mg for
adults, and 350 to 1,000 mg per day for children and young
people (depending on their age).

•Consider stone analysis for adults with ureteric or renal stones.
•Measure serum calcium for adults with ureteric or renal stones.
•Consider referring children and young people with ureteric or renal
stones to a paediatric nephrologist or paediatric urologist with
expertise in this area for assessment and metabolic investigations

NICE Guidelines (2019)

14.2 Case 1

The case

- 55 year old male
- Impacted distal 1cm left ureteric stone – present for greater than 2 months.
- Concurrent left inter pole stone in a long tight infundibulum.
- Hostile distal left ureter.
- Prior radiotherapy to prostate for prostate cancer.

The condition

- 9 mm left interpolar calculus and 7 mm left distal ureteric calculus.

Pre-operative imaging

- CT KUB
- Prior pyelogram
- Figures 14.1, 14.2, 14.3 for preoperative imaging and Fig. 14.4 for access to a renal pelvic stone with distal ureteric stone

The equipment

- Sensor wire 0.08 Fr-   nitinol core over a hydrophilic coating
- Ureteric catheter- white (soft) or blue (stiffer)
- Contrast- Urograffin 150 or 300.
- Long rigid ureteroscope
- Flexible ureteroscope
- Access sheath

The strategy

- Rigid cystoscope in, with bridge
- Change to biopsy forceps
- Pass sensor to renal pelvis, screen stent out
- Do a retrograde to see whether there are stones in the ureter
- Using the long rigid, clear the ureteric stones 1st.
- Laser and clear lower pole stones
- Fragment and extract, start at 0.5/5 on laser settings
- 6x24 fr stent

The difficulties

- Left URETEROSCOPY + laser fragmentation of residual ureteric stone and attempted flexible URS- PINHOLE and very difficult - dilated area just proximal to intramural ureter.
- Here sat further stones- fragmented and extracted
- 2cm strictured area on retrograde
- 8 French Rocomed silicone stent

The outcome

- Stones fully cleared from kidney.
- Chase stone type.
- Stent register- tract stent and ensure it is removed.
- Dietary advice including BAUS information leaflet- recurrent stone former in high risk stone category.
- TFTs, Calcium, Urate .

Ureteric strictures and stones
Ureteroscopic management has supplanted shockwave lithotripsy as the most common treatment of upper tract stone disease.
Thirty-eight patients with 40 ureteral strictures following URS for upper tract stone disease were identified. (May, 20090

Thirty-five percent of patients had hydronephrosis or known stone impaction at the time of initial URS (May, 2009)
After stricture diagnosis, the mean number of procedures requiring sedation or general anaesthesia performed for stricture management was 3.3 ± 1.8 (range 1-10).

Eleven strictures (27.5%) were successfully managed with endoscopic techniques alone, 37.5% underwent reconstruction, 10% had a chronic stent/nephrostomy, and 10 (25%) required nephrectomy (May 2009)
The surgical morbidity of ureteral strictures incurred following ureteroscopy for stone disease can be severe, with a low success rate of endoscopic management and a high procedural burden that may lead to nephrectomy (May, 2009).

Fig. 14.1 Left sided pyelogram

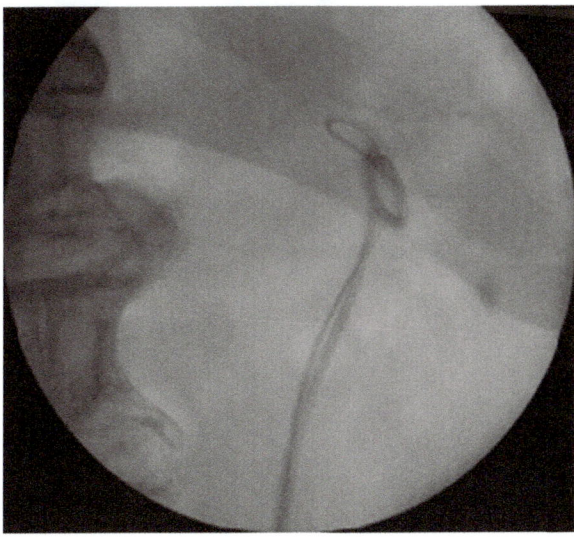

Fig. 14.2 Pre-operative
CT

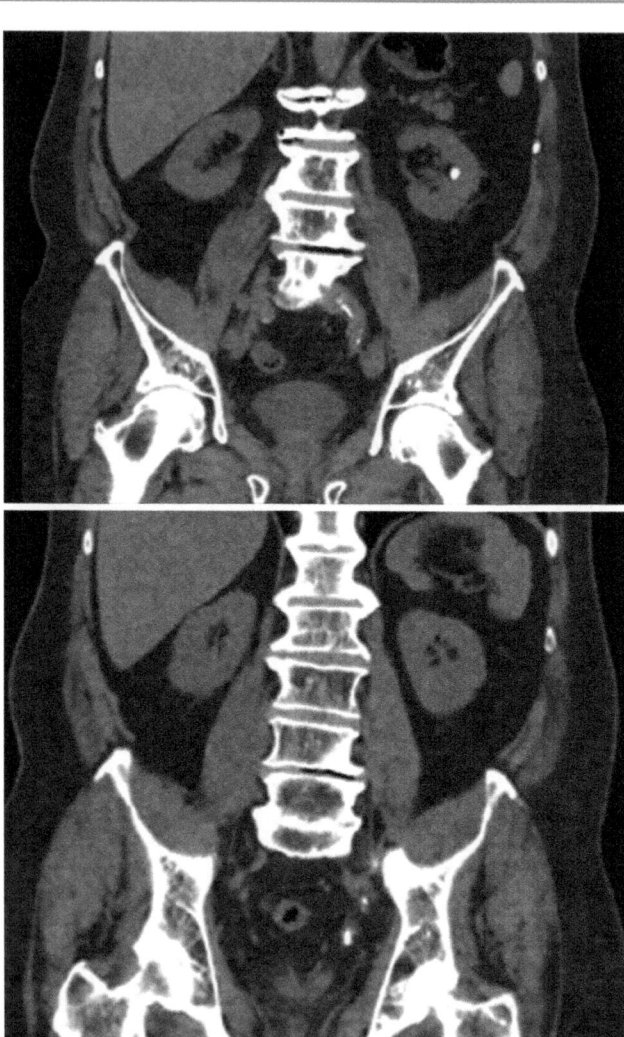

Fig. 14.3 Stricture on retrograde

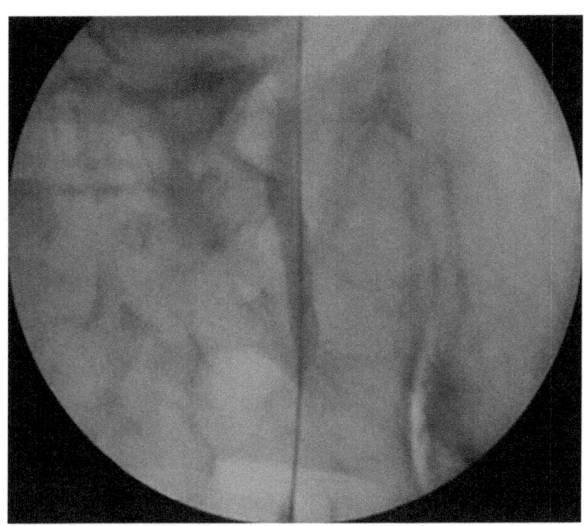

Fig. 14.4 Access to renal pelvic stone with a distal ureteric stone

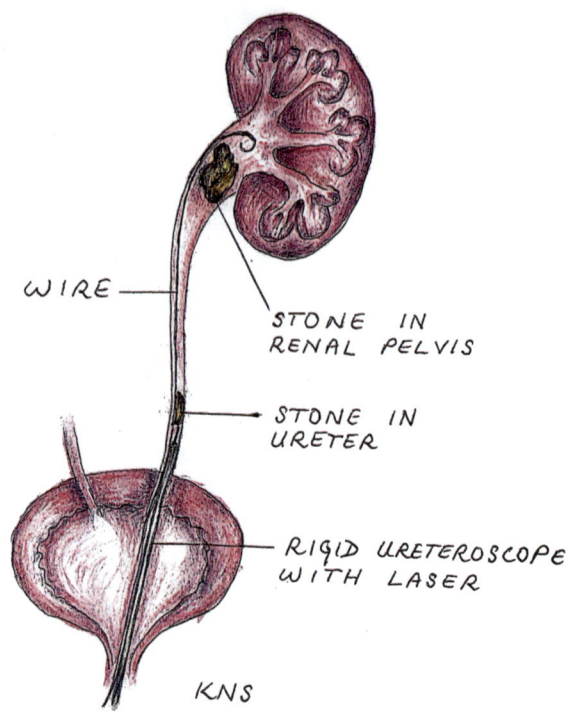

14.3   Case 2

The case

- 76 year old male
- Bilateral hydronephrosis
- Multiple bilateral renal calc
- Nodular prostate
- PSA 19
- Pacemaker (for AF), usually on warfarin, INR currently 1.4

The condition

- Left 2x1mm renal stones- midpole? Randalls plaques
- Right – 8mm, 5mm midpole stones, 9mm distal ureter

Pre-operative imaging

- CT KUB
- Prior pyelogram
- (Figs. 14.5, 14.6, 14.7 and 14.8)

The equipment

- Sensor wire 0.08 Fr- nitinol core over a hydrophilic coating
- Ureteric catheter- white (soft) or blue (stiffer)
- Contrast- Urograffin 150 or 300.
- Long rigid ureteroscope
- Flexible ureteroscope
- Access sheath

The strategy

- Rigid cystoscope in, with bridge
- Change to biopsy forceps
- Pass sensor to renal pelvis, screen stent out
- Do a retrograde to see whether there are stones in the ureter
- Using the long rigid, clear the ureteric stones 1st.
- Laser and clear lower pole stones
- Fragment and extract, start at 0.5/5 on laser settings
- 6x24 fr stent

The difficulties

- Right URETEROSCOPY + laser fragmentation of residual ureteric stone and attempted flexible URS- strictured and kinked and very difficult - dilated area just proximal to intra-mural ureter- use nottingham ilators.
- 2cm strictured area on retrograde
- 8 French hydrophillic stent used to see if stricture would open

The outcome

- Stones fully cleared from kidney.
- Chase stone type.
- Stent register- tract stent and ensure it is removed.
- Dietary advice including BAUS information leaflet- recurrent stone former in high risk stone category.
- Once stent removed, MAG 3 renogram to see if kidney was obstructed.
- TFTs, Calcium, Urate.

Fig. 14.5 CT KUB
demonstrating stones

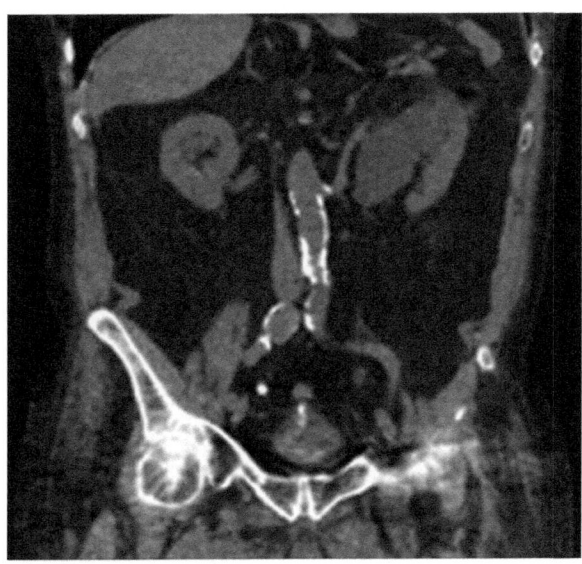

Fig. 14.6 CT KUB
demonstrating renal stones
and bilateral stents

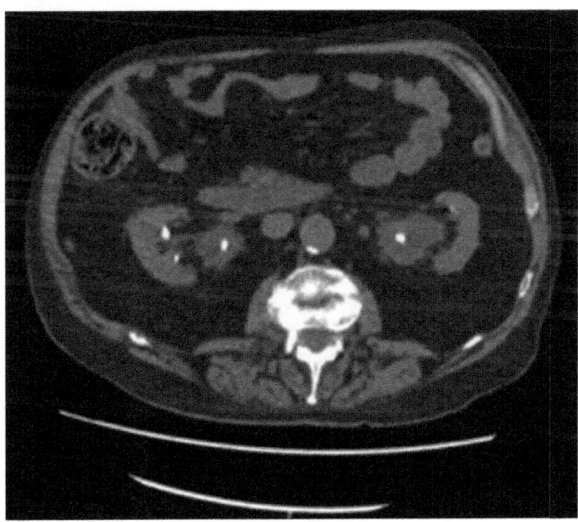

Fig. 14.7 Kinked ureter
from prior retrograde that
may be obstructing stone

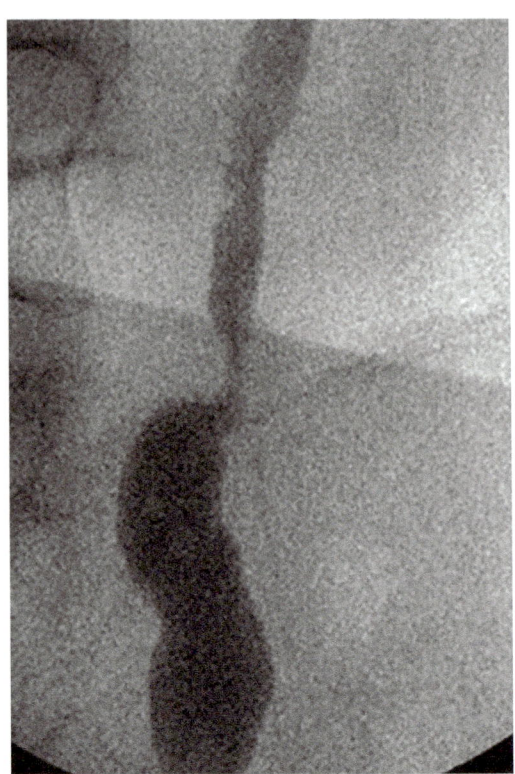

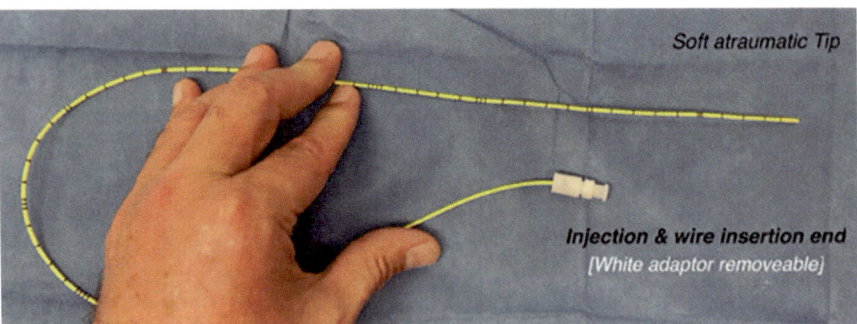

Soft atraumatic Tip

Injection & wire insertion end
[White adaptor removeable]

Fig. 14.8 A Ureteric catheter- used to do the retrograde

14.4   Case 3

The case
- 45 year old female
- Recurrent stone former
- Awaiting parathyroidectomy

The condition
- 6mm distal left ureteric stone
- Multiple bilateral renal stones with nephrocalcinosis
- 15 renal stones in total

Pre-operative imaging
- CT KUB
- Prior pyelogram
- Figures 14.9, 14.10 and 14.11

The equipment

- Sensor wire 0.08 Fr- nitinol core over a hydrophilic coating
- Ureteric catheter- white (soft) or blue (stiffer)
- Contrast- Urograffin 150 or 300.
- Long (semi-rigid) rigid ureteroscope
- Flexible ureteroscope
- Access sheath

The strategy

- Rigid cystoscope in, with bridge
- Change to biopsy forceps
- Pass sensor to renal pelvis, screen stent out
- Do a retrograde to see whether there are stones in the ureter
- Using the long rigid, clear the ureteric stones 1st.
- Laser and clear lower pole stones
- Fragment and extract, start at 0.5/5 on laser settings
- 6x24 fr stent

The difficulties

- Left URETEROSCOPY + laser fragmentation of residual ureteric stone and attempted flexible URS- PINHOLE and very difficult - dilated area just proximal to intra-mural ureter.
- Here sat further stones- fragmented and extracted
- 2cm strictured area on retrograde
- 8 French Rocomed silicone stent

The outcome

- Stones fully cleared from kidney.
- Chase stone type
- Stent register- tract stent and ensure it is removed.
- Dietary advice including BAUS information leaflet- recurrent stone former in high risk stone category.
- TFTs, Calcium, Urate.

Morbidity of ureteric strictures
A well-known complication of endourological treatment for
impacted ureteral stones is the formation of ureteral strictures,
which has been reported to occur in 14.2% to 24% of cases (Xeng 2015).
Of the 77 patients who participated in the study, 5 developed
ureteral strictures. Thus, the stricture rate was 7.8% (Xeng 2015).

An analysis of the intraoperative risk factors including perforation
of the ureter, damage to the mucous membrane, and residual stone
impacted within the ureter mucosa revealed that none of these
factors contributed significantly to the formation of the ureteric
strictures (Xeng 2015).
The stone-related risk factors that were taken into consideration
were stone size, stone impaction site, and duration of impaction.
These stone factors also did not contribute significantly to the
formation of the ureteral strictures (Xeng 2015).

This prospective study failed to identify any predictable factors for
ureteral stricture formation. It is proposed that all patients undergo
a simple postoperative KUB ultrasound screening 3 months after
undergoing endoscopic treatment for impacted ureteral stones
(Xeng 2015).

Fig. 14.9 CT
demonstrating stone
burden

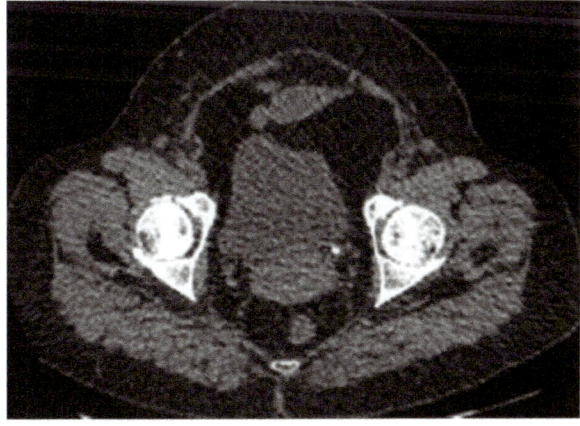

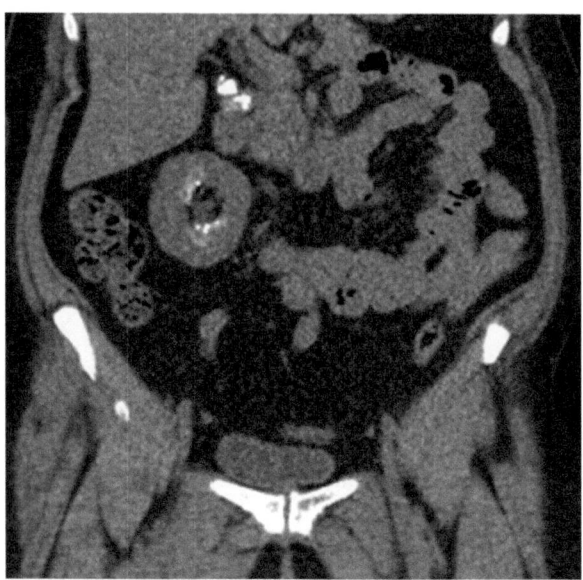

Fig. 14.10 CT demonstrating stone burden in kidneys

Fig. 14.11 Pyelogram on left kidney

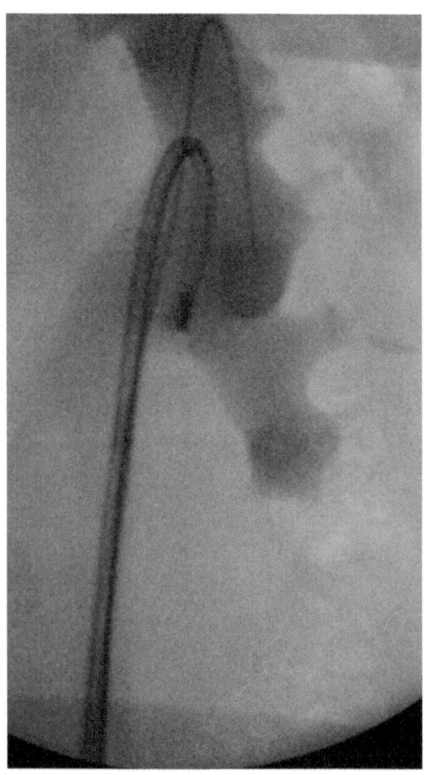

14.5 Patient Information and Consent

Why is this procedure being done?

- This procedure is being done to remove stone from the lower part of the tube from the kidney to the bladder
- This uses a camera through the bladder and stones are broken up using a laser
- This procedure is done with cameras to avoid more major operations such as open surgery for stone removal
- A stent will be required at the end of the procedure, which may be remove in a few days (stent on strings) or a couple of weeks using a camera (Flexible cystoscope)
- The procedure is done as a daycase and followup will be in at a routine outpatient appointment

What are the alternatives

- Conservative management
- ESWL- shock wave therapy to the stone to try and break it up- may require 2 sessions, f this fails, usually surgery is required
- Robotic or laparoscopic stone surgery- no commonly done for stones
- Open stone surgery- not commonly done for stones

What the procedure entails

- A general anaesthetic is used
- Antibiotics are given pre-procedure
- A camera is inserted and contrast studies are done
- A camera and laser will be passed to the kidney
- The stone will be broken to fragments or removed or dusted
- A stent will be passed up to the kidney that will be removed at a later date

The outcome

- Infection, sepsis, HDU/ ITU stay
- Bleeding
- Recurrence
- Remnant stone requiring further treatment
- Failure to reach stone requiring stenting and a 2nd look procedure or nephrostom
- Trauma to the ureter- abrasion, stricture, mucosal damage, ureteric reconstruction
- Anaesthetic risks - MI, CVA, PE, DVT, Chest infection

References

May PC, Hsi RS, Tran H, Stoller ML, Chew BH, Chi T, Usawachintachit M, Duty BD, Gore JL, Harper JD. The morbidity of ureteral strictures in patients with prior Ureteroscopic stone surgery: multi-institutional outcomes. J Endourol. 2018;32(4):309–14.

NICE Guideline. Renal and ureteric stones: assessment and management: NICE (2019) renal and ureteric stones: assessment and management. BJU Int. 2019 Feb;123(2):220–32.

Xeng Inn FAM, Singam P, Christopher-Chee-Kong HO, Sridharan R, HOD R, Bahadzor B, GOH EH, TAN GH, Zainuddin Z. Ureteral stricture formation after Ureteroscope treatment of impacted calculi: a prospective study. Korean J Urol. 2015;56(1):63–7.

Surgical Strategy for the Renal Pelvic Stone

15

15.1 Guidelines on Management of Renal Stones

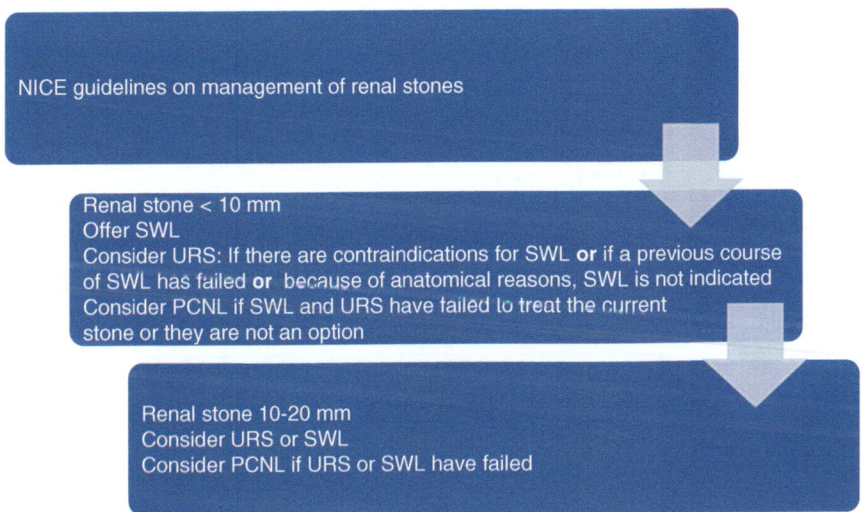

NICE guidelines on management of renal stones

Renal stone < 10 mm
Offer SWL
Consider URS: If there are contraindications for SWL **or** if a previous course of SWL has failed **or** because of anatomical reasons, SWL is not indicated
Consider PCNL if SWL and URS have failed to treat the current stone or they are not an option

Renal stone 10-20 mm
Consider URS or SWL
Consider PCNL if URS or SWL have failed

NICE Guidelines (2019)

Recommendations	Strength rating
Consider the stone composition before deciding on the method of removal, based on patient history, former stone analysis of the patient or Hounsfield unit (HU) on unenhanced computed tomography (CT).	Strong

© The Author(s), under exclusive license to Springer Nature
Switzerland AG 2021
S. S. Goonewardene et al., *Surgical Strategies in Endourology for Stone Disease*,
https://doi.org/10.1007/978-3-030-82143-2_15

Recommendations	Strength rating
Offer laparoscopic or open surgical stone removal in rare cases in which shock wave lithotripsy (SWL), retrograde or antegrade ureteroscopy and percutaneous nephrolithotomy fail, or are unlikely to be successful.	Strong

Türk et al. (2016)

15.2   Case 1

The case
- 75 year old female
- No information in records
- No letters from urology
- Admitted to A+E, fall and fever. Stone seen on scan. Hypothyroidism, depression, diabetes type II

The condition
- 14 mm left renal pelvic stone on CT

Pre-operative imaging
- CT KUB
- Fig 15.1

Pre-op surgical strategy
- Rigid cystoscope in, with bridge Figs. 15.2 and 15.3
- Change to biopsy forceps
- Pass sensor to renal pelvis, screen stent out
- Do a retrograde to see whether there are stones in the ureter
- Using the long rigid, clear the ureteric stones 1st.
- Laser and clear lower pole stones
- Fragment and extract, start at 0.5/5 on laser settings
- Be wary of using access sheath especially if ureter is friable and stone is impacted.
- 6x24 fr stent

The equipment

- Sensor wire 0.08 Fr- nitinol core over a hydrophilic coating
- Ureteric catheter- white (soft) or blue (stiffer)
- Contrast- Urograffin 150 or 300.
- Long rigid ureteroscope
- Flexible ureteroscope
- Access sheath

The strategy

- Rigid cystoscope in, with bridge
- Change to biopsy forceps
- Pass sensor to renal pelvis.
- Do a retrograde to see whether there are stones in the ureter
- Using the long rigid, do a diagnostic ureteroscopy to view all areas of the ureter
- Laserto stone
- If ureter clear identify renal pelvic stone. If in good position you may be able to laser with long rigid alone, but always have access sheath and flexible ureteroscopy on standby.
- Do not force the access sheath as the ureter can be tight
- 6x24 fr stent (female patient, shorter stent)

The difficulties

- Getting up past the stone sometimes the sensor won't pass
- If this happens, use the blue ureteric catheter, which will stiffen the guidewire, or a terumo wire (very hydrophilic)
- Once the wire is past the kink, get a lot of wire into the renal pelvis- the automatic reflex of wire is to straighten and straighten out the kink
- When passing up the long rigid ureteroscope, have a second wire as a probiscus to guide you.
- Poor vision- go for dusting over fragmentation.
- Use the washout technique to get rid of fragments

The outcome

- All examinations were negative, so patient did not require any further surgery e.g. nephrouretrectomy.
- A MAG 3 was conducted to ensure the kink was not causing obstruction.

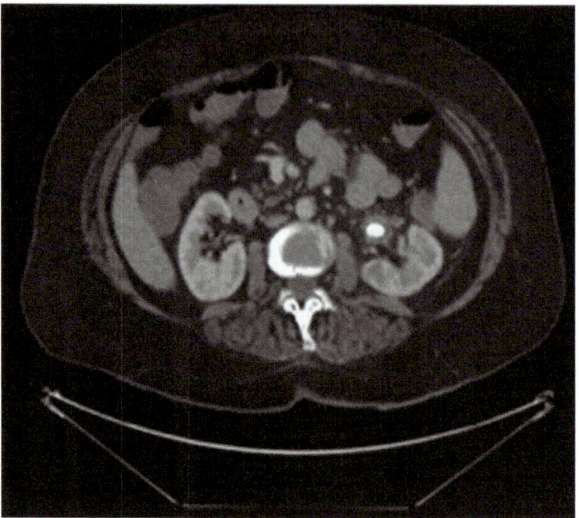

Fig. 15.1 CT scan demonstrating renal pelvic stone

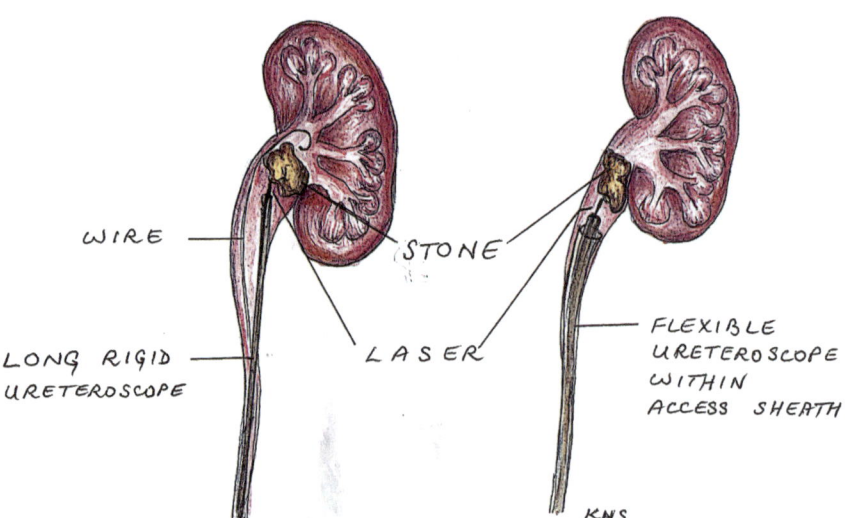

Fig. 15.2 Demonstrating management of renal pelvic stone

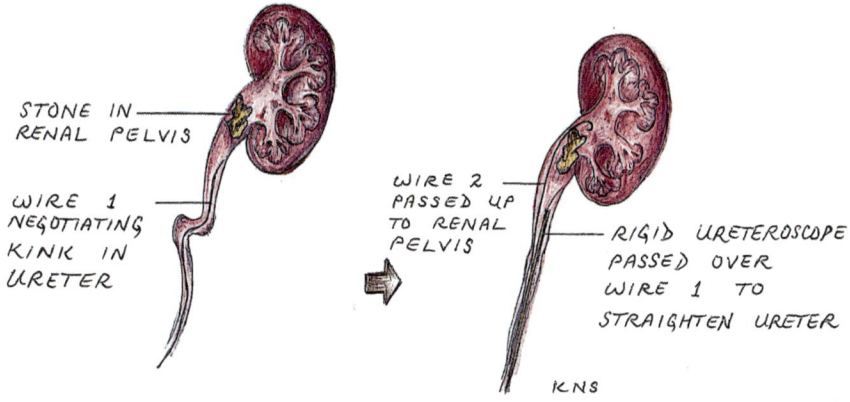

Fig. 15.3 Getting the wire past the kinked ureter

15.3   Supine vs. Prone PCNL Outcomes

Ozdemir, 2019 compared the outcomes of supine and prone miniaturized percutaneous nephrolithotomy (m-PNL) in the treatment of lower pole, middle pole and renal pelvic stones (Ozdemir, 2019).

The operation time and fluoroscopy time in supine m-PNL was significantly shorter than prone m-PNL group (58.1±45.9 vs. 80.1±40.0 min and 3.0±1.7 min vs. 4.9±4.5 min, p=0.025 and p=0.01, respectively) (Ozdemir, 2019). Overall and subgroup complication rates were comparable between groups (Ozdemir, 2019). There was no significant difference between the groups in terms of the success rates (supine m-PNL; 72.2%, prone m-PNL; 71.3%, p=0.902) (Ozdemir, 2019).

Supine m-PNL procedure is more advantageous in terms of operation time and fluoroscopy time in the treatment of lower pole, middle pole and renal pelvic stones (Ozdemir, 2019).

15.4   Points of Consent

Why is this procedure being done?

- This procedure is being done to remove stones from the renal pelvis of the kidney using a camera through the bladder
- Stones are broken up using a laser
- This procedure is done with cameras to avoid more major operations such as open surgery for stone removal
- A stent will be required at the end of the procedure, which may be removed in a few days (stent on strings) or a couple of weeks using a camera (Flexible cystoscope)

What are the alternatives

- Conservative management
- ESWL- shock wave therapy to the stone to try and break it up- may require 2 sessions, f this fails, usually surgery is required
- PCNL- using a camera through the back into the kidney, very large stones can be extracted
- Robotic or laparoscopic stone surgery- no commonly done for stones
- Open stone surgery- not common done for stones

What the procedure entails

- A general anaesthetic is used
- Antibiotics are given pre-procedure
- A camera is inserted and contrast studies are done
- A camera and laser will be passed to the kidney
- The stone will be broken to fragments or removed or dusted
- A stent will be passed up to the kidney that will be removed at a later date

The outcome

- Infection, sepsis, HDU/ ITU stay
- Bleeding
- Recurrence
- Remnant stone requiring further treatment
- Failure to reach stone requiring stenting and a 2nd look procedure or nephrostom
- Trauma to the ureter- abrasion, stricture, mucosal damage, ureteric reconstruction
- Anaesthetic risks - MI, CVA, PE, DVT, Chest infection

References

NICE Guideline. Renal and ureteric stones: assessment and management: NICE (2019) Renal and ureteric stones: assessment and management. BJU Int. Feb 2019;123(2):220–32.

Ozdemir H, Erbin A, Sahan M, Savun M, Cubuk A, Yazici O, Akbulut MF, Sarilar O. Comparison of supine and prone miniaturized percutaneous Nephrolithotomy in the treatment of lower pole, middle pole and renal pelvic stones: a matched pair analysis. Int Braz J Urol. 2019;45(5):956–64.

Türk C, Petřík A, Sarica K, Seitz C, Skolarikos A, Straub M. Thomas Knoll EAU guidelines on interventional treatment for urolithiasis. Eur Urol. 2016;69(3):475–82.

Surgical Strategies in PUJ Obstruction

16

16.1 PUJO-Preoperative Evaluation, Surgical Management, Exclusion Criteria

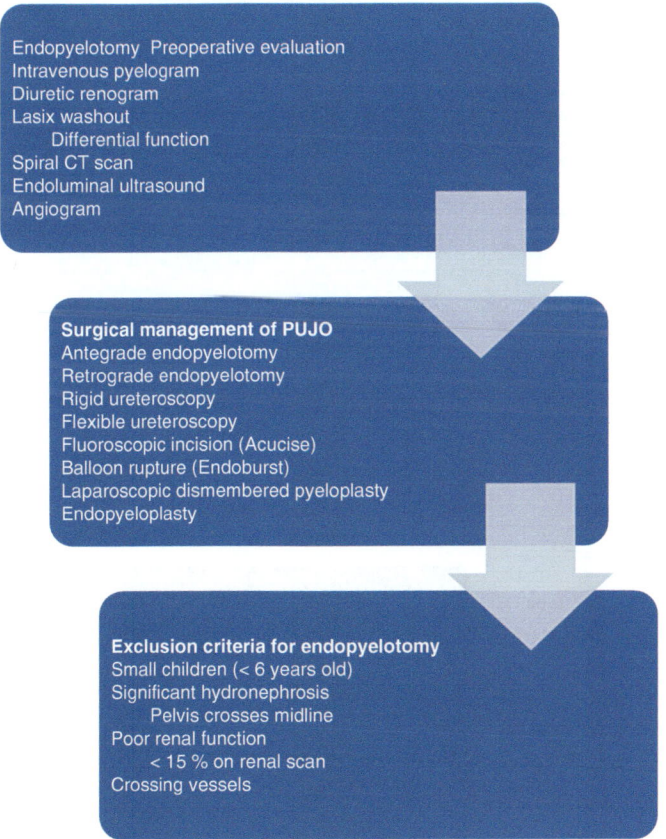

Endopyelotomy Preoperative evaluation
Intravenous pyelogram
Diuretic renogram
Lasix washout
    Differential function
Spiral CT scan
Endoluminal ultrasound
Angiogram

Surgical management of PUJO
Antegrade endopyelotomy
Retrograde endopyelotomy
Rigid ureteroscopy
Flexible ureteroscopy
Fluoroscopic incision (Acucise)
Balloon rupture (Endoburst)
Laparoscopic dismembered pyeloplasty
Endopyeloplasty

Exclusion criteria for endopyelotomy
Small children (< 6 years old)
Significant hydronephrosis
    Pelvis crosses midline
Poor renal function
    < 15 % on renal scan
Crossing vessels

16.2   Antegrade Endopyelotomy

Antegrade endopyelotomy
Introduced by Wickham in 1984 and popularized by Smith
Percutaneous access to renal pelvis
Lateral incision under direct vision
Full thickness incision
Stent placement (for 6 weeks) (Fig. 16.1)

Results for antegrade endopyelotomy
n=401
Follow-up   51 months (6-144 mo)
Overall success rate   85%
1^0 UPJ success   82%
2^0 UPJ success   89%
Gupta & Smith, 1997

Hydronephrosis - Success
        Grade 2   96%
        Grade 4   50%
Renal function - Success
        Good   92%
        Moderate   80%
        Poor   54%
Crossing vessels impact successful outcome
in only 4% of patients
Gupta & Smith, 1997

Fig. 16.1 Antegrade
endopyelotomy

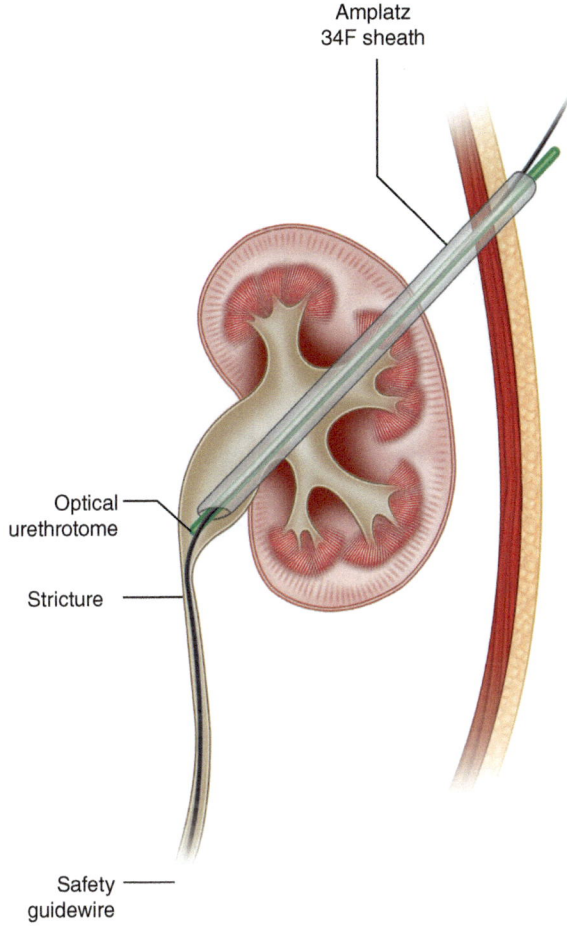

Amplatz
34F sheath

Optical
urethrotome

Stricture

Safety
guidewire

Antegrade endopyelotomy

16.3   Puncture, Method of Incision

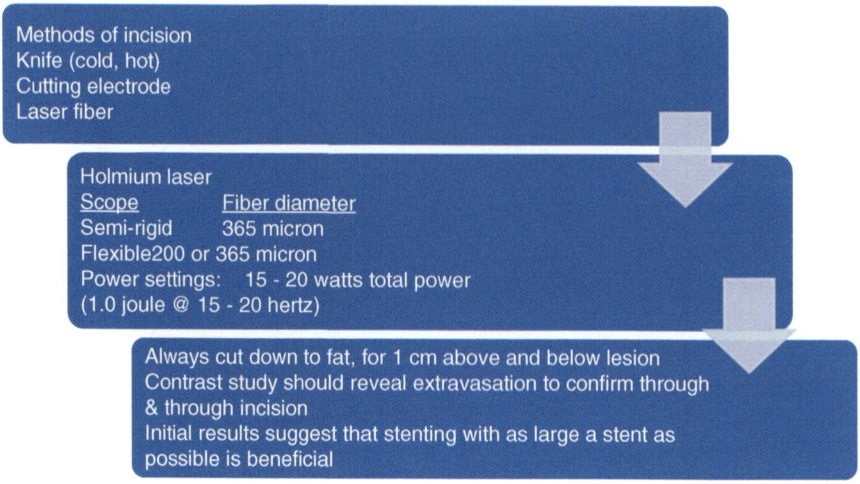

Methods of incision
Knife (cold, hot)
Cutting electrode
Laser fiber

Holmium laser
Scope   Fiber diameter
Semi-rigid   365 micron
Flexible200 or 365 micron
Power settings: 15 - 20 watts total power
(1.0 joule @ 15 - 20 hertz)

Always cut down to fat, for 1 cm above and below lesion
Contrast study should reveal extravasation to confirm through
& through incision
Initial results suggest that stenting with as large a stent as
possible is beneficial

Figures 16.2 and 16.3 for method of incision and skin to calyx distance.

Fig. 16.2 Method of approach-mid, upper or lower calyx

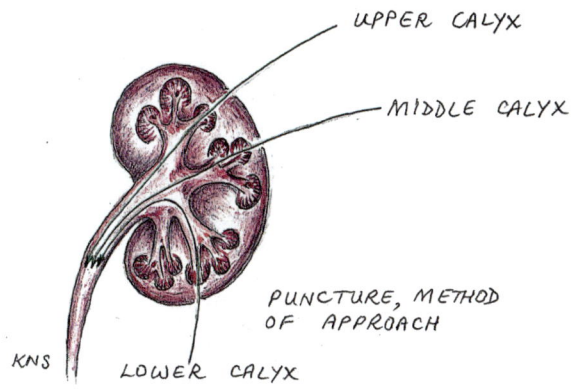

Fig. 16.3 Aim to cross the shortest distance to enter each calyx

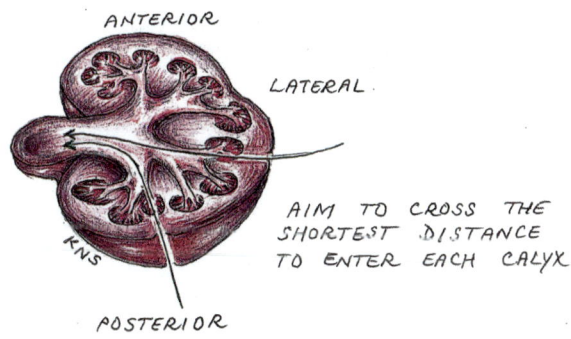

16.4   Retrograde Ureteroscopic Endopyelotomy

Operating time200 minutes
Incision   2 F, 3 F, 5 F
Hospital stay   4.5 days
Stent duration   6 weeks
(Clayman, 1990)

Direct visualization with ureteroscope
Incision with holmium laser or electrocautery
Balloon dilatation to 24 Fr
Placement of stent

Follow-up   12 months (5-24 mo)
Asymptomati   80%
IVP
Improved   3
Unchanged   2
Renal scan
Normal   5
Prolonged   2
Complications
Ureteral stricture   20%
(Clayman, 1990)

Follow-up   62 months (28-146 mo)
Overall success rate   78%
Average treatment time   90 min
Outpatient procedure   56%
(Thomas, 1996)

16.5   Comparison of Antegrade and Retrograde Approaches

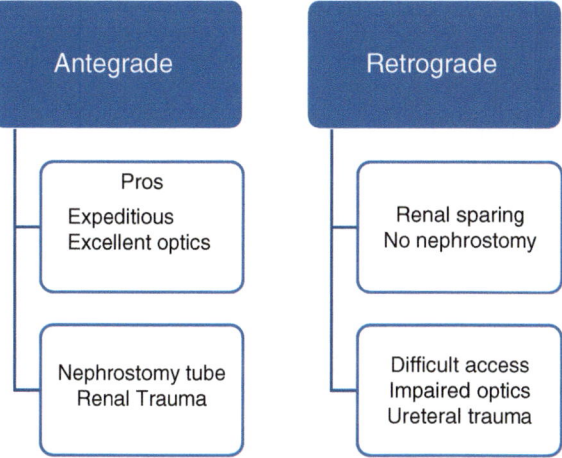

16.6   Cutting Dilation Endopyelotomy

Follow-up   22 months (14-29 mo)
Overall success rate   78%
1^0 UPJ success   71%
2^0 UPJ success   100%
75 % of failures occurred within the first 4 months
(Cohen, et al, 1997)

16.7   Outcomes from Endopyelotomy

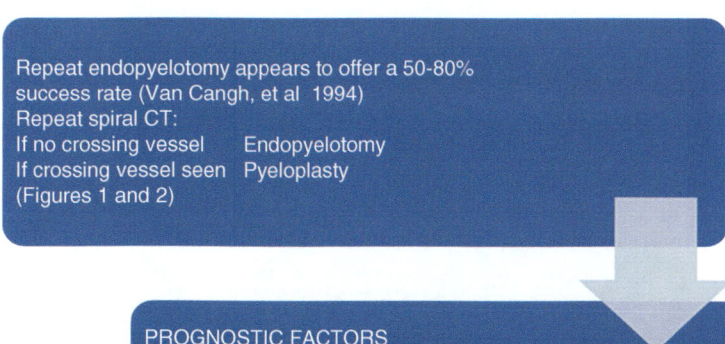

Repeat endopyelotomy appears to offer a 50-80%
success rate (Van Cangh, et al 1994)
Repeat spiral CT:
If no crossing vessel   Endopyelotomy
If crossing vessel seen   Pyeloplasty
(Figures 1 and 2)

PROGNOSTIC FACTORS
102 consecutive endopyelotomy pts, f/u 5 yrs
Digital angiogram
        Crossing vessels
Diuretic IVP
        Hydronephrosis (grades 1 - 4)
(Van Cangh, et al 1994)

Figures 16.4 and 16.5 below for success rates for Endopyelotomy and outcomes.

Degree of Hydronephrosis	Massive	Severe	Moderate			
	36%	86%	96%			

Jabbour & Smith, 1998

Fig. 16.4   Success rates from Endopyelotomy (Jabbour et al. 1998)

Renal function	<25%	25.40%	>40%	
Success rates	57%	86%	90%	

Jabbour & Smith, 1998

Fig. 16.5   Outcomes depending on renal function (Jabbour et al. 1998)

16.8   Crossing Vessels

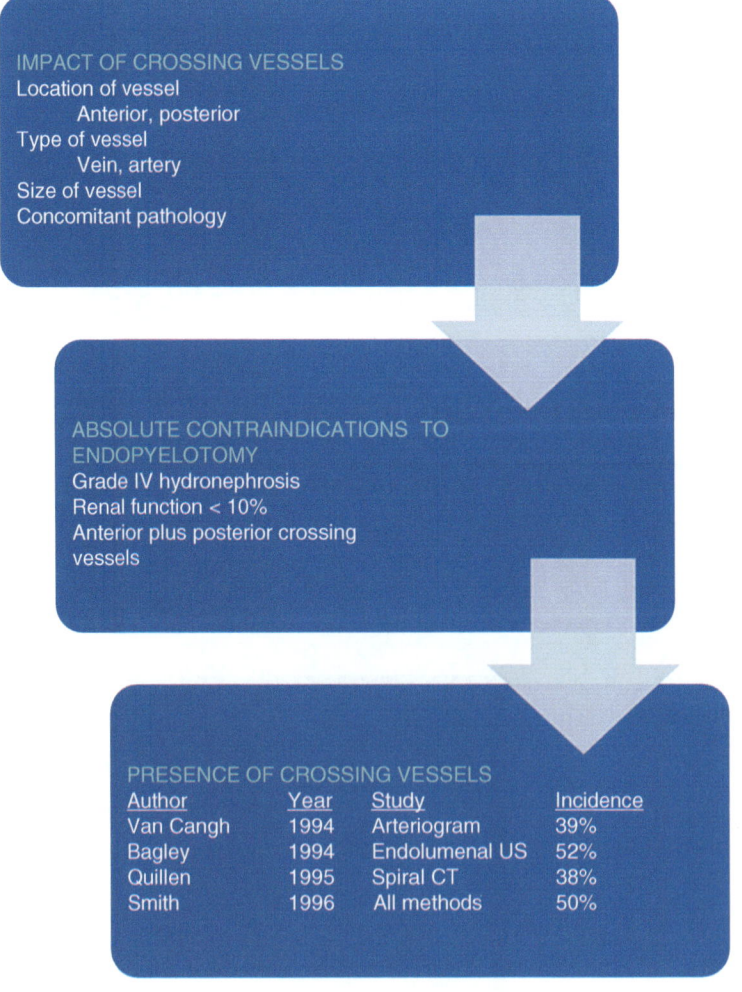

16.9   PUJO Recommendations

Endopyelotomy (Endoscopic / Acucise)
Normal-sized renal pelvis
Failed pyeloplasty
Secondary UPJ obstruction

Laparoscopic / Open/Robotic Pyeloplasty
Unusual ureteral insertion
"Crossing" vessel
Reduction pyeloplasty

16.10   Mag 3 Renogram Vs. Isotope Renogram in Functional PUJ Outcomes

Turk evaluated and compared the diagnostic accuracy of dynamic contrast-enhanced magnetic resonance imaging (dMRI) and isotope renogram in the functional evaluation of pelviureteric junction obstruction (PUJO) (Turk, 2018). Of 33 patients taken up for surgical intervention, 12 underwent laparoscopic nephrectomy and 21 of them pyeloplasty. The mean glomerular filtration rates (GFRs) as measured by isotope renogram and dMRI were 22.5+4.2 mL/min and 23.8+3.1 mL/min respectively (Turk, 2018).

The calculation of GFR by isotope renogram, showed good correlation with that of dMRI with correlation coefficient of 0.93 (Turk, 2018). The dMRI was able to reveal the functional status of the renal unit accurately. dMRI did not yield false positive results with 20 of 21 patients scheduled for pyeloplasty and 11 of 12 patients scheduled for nephrectomy (Turk, 2018). Isotope renogram had a false positive result in 3 cases compared with surgical diagnosis.

Analysis of renal function using dMRI yielded results comparable to those of renal scintigraphy, with superior spatial and contrast resolution (Turk, 2018). It was also better in prompting management decisions with respect to the obstructed systems. dMRI can be used as a "one stop imaging examination" that can replace different imaging methods used for morphological, etiological and functional evaluation of PUJO (Turk, 2018).

References

Bagley DH, Liu JB, Grasso M, Goldberg BB. Endoluminal sonography in evaluation of the obstructed ureteropelvic junction. J Endourol. 1998;8(4):287–92.

Clayman RV, Basler JW, Kavoussi L, Picus DD. Ureteronephroscopic endopyelotomy. J Urol. 144(2 Pt 1):246–51.

Gupta M, Smith D. Open surgical exploration after failed endopyelotomy: a 12-year perspective. J Urol. 1997;157(5):1613–9.

Jabbour ME, Goldfischer ER, Klima WJ, Stravodimos KG, Smith AD. Endopyelotomy after failed pyeloplasty: the long-term results. J Urol. 1998;160(3 Pt 1):690–3.

Sivakumar VN, Indiran V, Sathyanathan BP. Dynamic MRI and isotope renogram in the functional evaluation of pelviureteric junction obstruction: a comparative study. Turk J Urol. 2018;44(1):45–50.

Thomas R, Monga M, Klein EW. Ureteroscopic retrograde endopyelotomy for management of ureteropelvic junction obstruction. J Endourol. 1996;10(2):141–5.

Van Cangh PJ, Wese FX, Opsomer R, Pirson Y, Squifflet JP. Urologic complications of renal transplantation. Acta Urol Belg. 1994;62(4):1–14.

Surgical Strategy for Proximal Ureteric Stone

17

17.1 Guidelines on Proximal Ureteric Stones

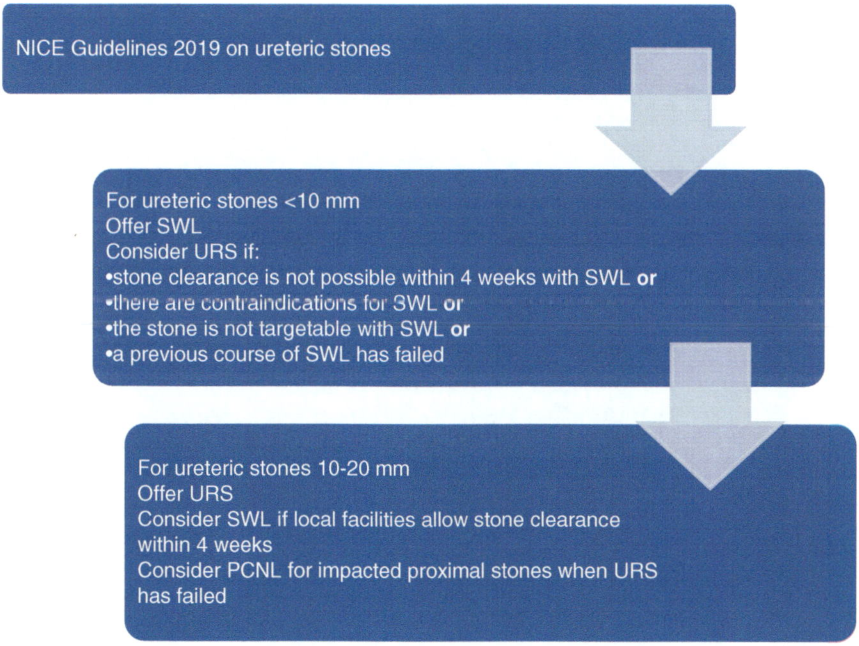

NICE Guidelines 2019 on ureteric stones
For ureteric stones <10 mm
Offer SWL
Consider URS if:
•stone clearance is not possible within 4 weeks with SWL **or**
•there are contraindications for SWL **or**
•the stone is not targetable with SWL **or**
•a previous course of SWL has failed
For ureteric stones 10-20 mm
Offer URS
Consider SWL if local facilities allow stone clearance within 4 weeks
Consider PCNL for impacted proximal stones when URS has failed

S. S. Goonewardene et al., *Surgical Strategies in Endourology for Stone Disease*, https://doi.org/10.1007/978-3-030-82143-2_17

17.2   Role of ESWL in Proximal Ureteric Stones

EAU Guidelines on ESWL, 2019

Summary of evidence and guidelines for SWL

Summary of evidence	LE
Proper acoustic coupling between the cushion of the treatment head and the patient's skin is important	2
Careful imaging control of localisation of stone contributes to outcome of treatment	2a
Careful control of pain during treatment is necessary to limit pain-induced movements and excessive respiratory excursions	1a
Antibiotic prophylaxis is recommended in the case of internal stent placement, infected stones or bacteriuria	1a

ESWL can be used for proximal ureteric stones, as long as there is no evidence of obstruction, sepsis or AKI.

Shock wave lithotripsy (SWL) is a well - established treatment option for urolithiasis (Lingeman, 2016). The technology of SWL has undergone significant changes in an attempt to better optimize the results while reducing failure rates. There are some important limitations that restrict the use of SWL (Lingeman, 2016).

Efficacy has been shown to vary between lithotripters (Lingeman, 2016). Factors to consider in proper patient selection include skin - to - stone distance and stone size (Lingeman, 2016). Careful attention to the rate of shock wave administration and proper coupling of the treatment head to the patient have important influences on the success of lithotripsy (Lingeman, 2016).

Proper selection of patients who are expected to respond well to SWL, as well as attention to the technical aspects of the procedure are the keys to SWL success (Lingeman, 2016). Studies aiming to determine the mechanisms of shock wave action in stone breakage have begun to suggest new treatment strategies to improve success rates and safety (Lingeman, 2016).

17.3   Case 1

The case
- 50 year old female
- Emergency stenting.
- Admitted with renal colic from A+E
- Unable to get up to stone at time of stenting
- 8x24 stent in situ

The condition
- 15 mm proximal right ureteric stone

Pre-operative imaging
- CT KUB, pyelogram from prior stenting
- Figures 17.1 and 17.2

Pre-op surgical strategy
- Rigid cystoscope in, with bridge
- Pass sensor to renal pelvis, screen stent out
- Do a retrograde to see whether there are stones in the ureter
- Using the long rigid, clear the ureteric stone
- Aim to dust due to stone burden
- Fragment and extract, start at 0.4J/10Hz on laser settings
- Be wary of using access sheath especially if ureter is friable and stone is impacted.
- 7 fr multilength

The equipment

- Sensor wire 0.08 Fr- nitinol core over a hydrophilic coating
- (Have the Terumo wire, and Reo Tracer wire on Standby)
- Ureteric catheter- white (soft) or blue (stiffer)
- Contrast- Urograffin 150 or 300.
- Long rigid ureteroscope
- Flexible ureteroscope, Access sheath on standby

The strategy

- Rigid cystoscope in, with bridge
- Pass sensor to renal pelvis.
- Do a retrograde to see whether there are stones in the ureter
- Using the long rigid, do a diagnostic ureteroscopy to view all areas of the ureter
- Laser to stone
- If ureter clear identify renal pelvic stone. If in a good position you may be able to laser with long rigid alone, but always have access sheath and flexible ureteroscopy on standby.
- Do not force the access sheath as the ureter can be tight- aim to dust and clear stone
- 6x24 fr stent (female patient, shorter stent)

The difficulties

- Getting up past the stone sometimes the sensor won't pass
- If this happens, use the blue ureteric catheter, which will stiffen the guidewire, or a terumo wire (very hydrophilic)
- Once the wire is past the kink, get a lot of wire into the renal pelvis- the automatic reflex of wire is to straighten and straighten out the kink.
- When passing up the long rigid ureteroscope, have a second wire as a probiscus to guide you.
- Poor vision- go for dusting over fragmentation.
- Use the washout technique to get rid of fragments

The outcome

- All examinations were negative, so patient did not require any further surgery e.g. nephrouretrectomy
- A MAG 3 was conducted to ensure the kink was not causing obstruction.

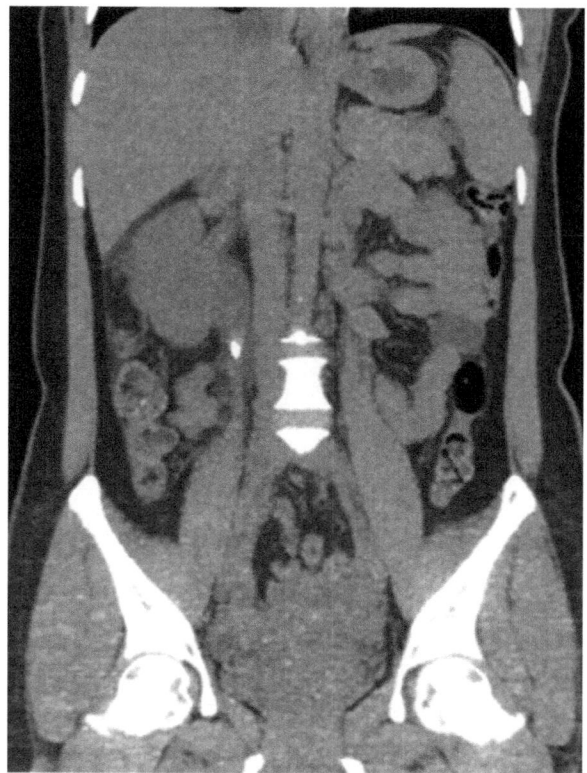

Fig. 17.1 Right proximal ureteric stone

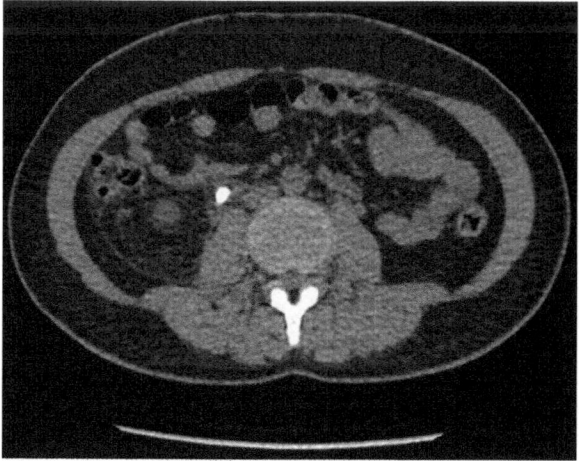

Fig. 17.2 Right proximal ureteric stone

Figures 17.3 and 17.4 demonstrating operative strategy to right proximal ureteric stone and a MAG 3 renogram.

Fig. 17.3 Demonstrating approach and access to a right proximal ureteric stone

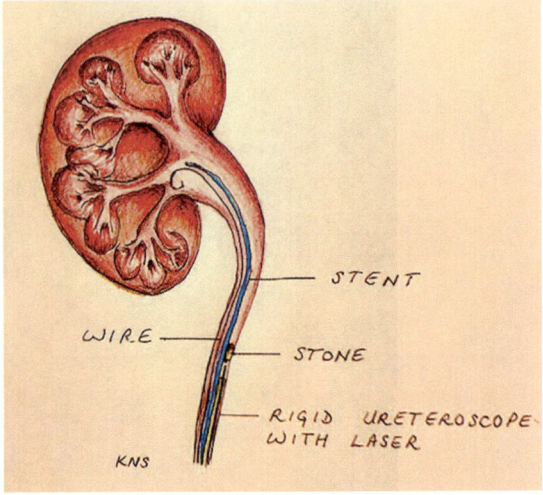

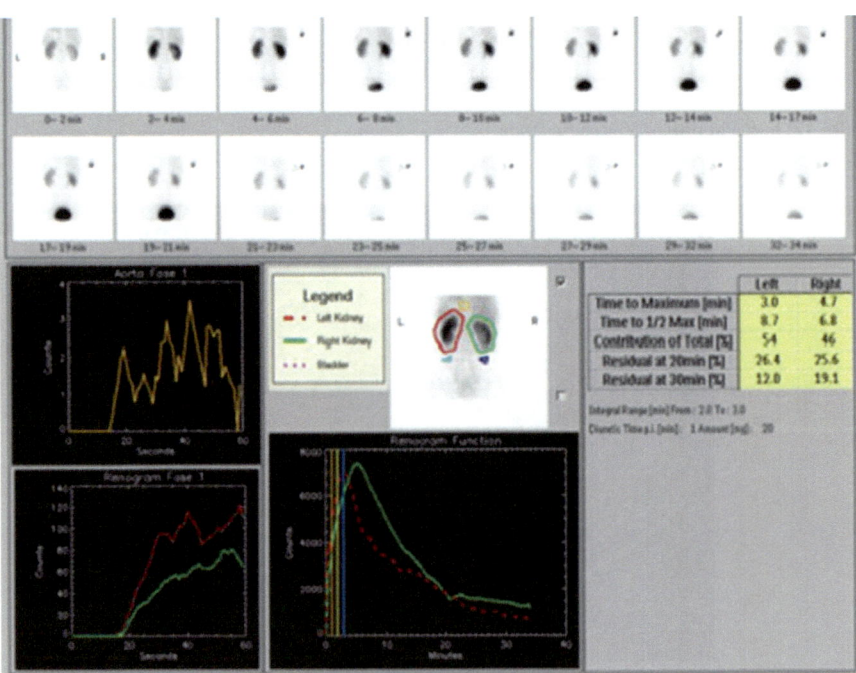

Fig. 17.4 A type 1 curve on MAG 3 renogram- demonstrating good drainage of both kidneys and no evidence of stricture

17.4   Patient Information and Consent

Why is this procedure being done?

- This procedure is being done to remove stones from the top part of the ureter using a camera through the bladder
- Stones are broken up using a laser
- This procedure is done with cameras to avoid more major operations such as open surgery for stone removal
- A stent will be required at the end of the procedure, which may be removed in a few days (stent on strings) or a couple of weeks using a camera (flexible cystoscope)
- The procedure is done as a daycase and followup will be in at a routine outpatient appointment

What are the alternatives

- Conservative management
- ESWL- shock wave therapy to the stone to try and break it up- may require 2 sessions, f this fails, usually surgery is required
- PCNL- using a camera through the back into the kidney, very large stones can be extracted
- Robotic or laparoscopic stone surgery- no commonly done for stones
- Open stone surgery- not commonly done for stones

What the procedure entails

- A general anaesthetic is used
- Antibiotics are given pre-procedure
- A camera is inserted and contrast studies are done
- A camera and laser will be passed to the kidney
- The stone will be broken to fragments or removed or dusted
- A stent will be passed up to the kidney that will be removed at a later date

The outcome

- Infection, sepsis, HDU/ ITU stay
- Bleeding
- Recurrence
- Remnant stone requiring further treatment
- Failure to reach stone requiring stenting and a 2nd look procedure or nephrostomy
- Trauma to the ureter- abrasion, stricture, mucosal damage, ureteric reconstruction
- Anaesthetic risks - MI, CVA, PE, DVT, Chest infection

References

Desai M, Sun Y, Buchholz N, Fuller A, Matsuda T, Matlaga B, Miller N, Bolton D, Alomar M, Ganpule A. Treatment selection for urolithiasis: percutaneous nephrolithomy, ureteroscopy, shock wave lithotripsy, and active monitoring. World J Urol. 2017;35(9):1395–9.

Elmansy HE, Lingeman JE. Recent advances in lithotripsy technology and treatment strategies: a systematic review update. Int J Surg. 2016;36(Pt D):676–80.

NICE Guideline – Renal and Ureteric Stones: Assessment and Management: NICE. Renal and ureteric stones: assessment and management. BJU Int. 2019;123(2): 220–32.

Türk C, Skolarikos A, Neisius A, Petřík A, Seitz C, Thomas K, Guidelines Associates, Donaldson JF, Drake T, Grivas N, Ruhayel Y. EAU guidelines, urolithiasis, 2019.

Surgical Strategy for VUJ Stones

18.1　Guidelines on Ureteric Stones

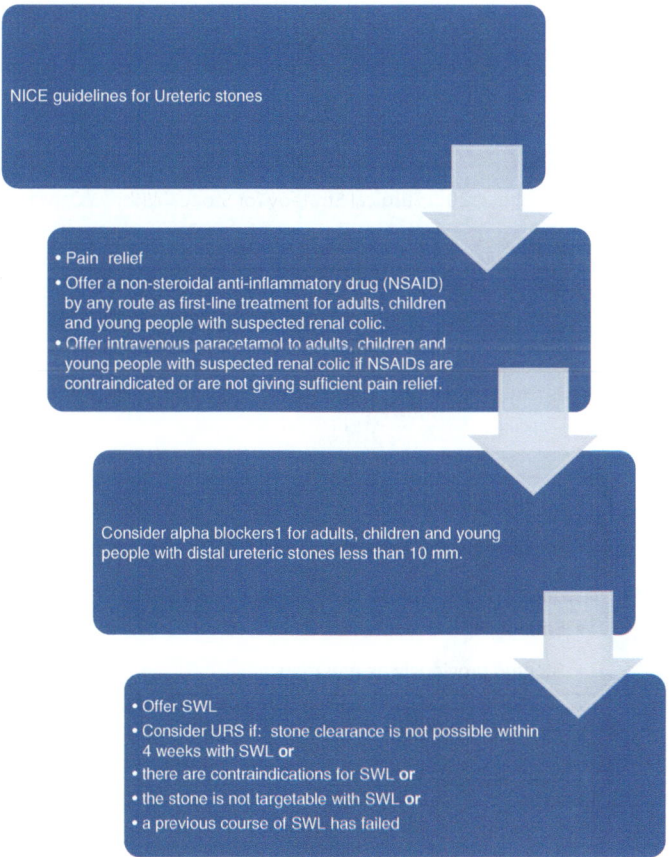

NICE guidelines for Ureteric stones

- Pain relief
- Offer a non-steroidal anti-inflammatory drug (NSAID) by any route as first-line treatment for adults, children and young people with suspected renal colic.
- Offer intravenous paracetamol to adults, children and young people with suspected renal colic if NSAIDs are contraindicated or are not giving sufficient pain relief.

Consider alpha blockers1 for adults, children and young people with distal ureteric stones less than 10 mm.

- Offer SWL
- Consider URS if: stone clearance is not possible within 4 weeks with SWL **or**
- there are contraindications for SWL **or**
- the stone is not targetable with SWL **or**
- a previous course of SWL has failed

NICE Guidelines, 2019

© The Author(s), under exclusive license to Springer Nature
Switzerland AG 2021
S. S. Goonewardene et al., *Surgical Strategies in Endourology for Stone Disease*,
https://doi.org/10.1007/978-3-030-82143-2_18

18.2   Medical Expulsive Therapy and Ureteric Stones

The Suspend Trial - medical expulsive therapy for
ureteric stones (Pickard, 2015)

Pickard examined treatment with the muscle-relaxant
drugs tamsulosin hydrochloride (Petyme, TEVA UK Ltd)
and nifedipine (Coracten(®), UCB Pharma Ltd) as
medical expulsive therapy (MET) for passage of
ureteric stones.

 The proportion of participants who spontaneously
passed their stone did not differ between MET and
placebo or between tamsulosin and nifedipine.

These findings were unchanged by extensive sensitivity
analyses around predictors of stone passage, including
sex, stone size and stone location.

Tamsulosin and nifedipine did not increase the likelihood of
stone passage over 4 weeks for people with ureteric colic,
and use of these drugs is very unlikely to be cost-effective for
the NHS.

Further work is required to investigate the phenomenon of
large, high-quality trials showing smaller effect size than
meta-analysis of several small, lower-quality studies.

18.3   Case 1

The case
- 50 year old female
- Recurrent stone former

The condition
- 5mm right VUJ stone
- Stented previously as emergency

Pre-operative imaging
- CT KUB
- Prior pyelogram

The

- Sensor wire 0.08 Fr- nitinol core over a hydrophilic coating
- Ureteric catheter- white (soft) or blue (stiffer)
- Contrast- Urograffin 150 or 300.
- Long rigid ureteroscope
- Flexible ureteroscope, Access sheath on standby

The strategy

- Get the sensor wire up to kidney (Fig. 18.1)
- Rigid cystoscope in, with bridge
- Change to biopsy forceps
- Screen stent out, and pass sensor to renal pelvis
- Do a retrograde to see whether there are stones in the ureter
- Using the long rigid, clear the ureteric stone.
- Put zero tip basket behind stone, and laser stone.
- Fragment and extract, start at 0.4/10 on laser settings
- 6x24 fr stent

The difficulties

- The stone can often fly to the kidey
- Flexion of the flexible cystoscopy to see the stone
- Stone must be repositioned in the a midpole calyx, this is a better position for fragmention
- Properly clearing stone, which may be in a dependant position.

The outcome

- Stones fully cleared from kidney.
- Chase stone type.
- Stent register- tract stent and ensure it is removed.
- Dietary advice including BAUS information leaflet.
- TFTs, Calcium, Urate.

Fig. 18.1 Getting a sensor
wire past a VUJ stone

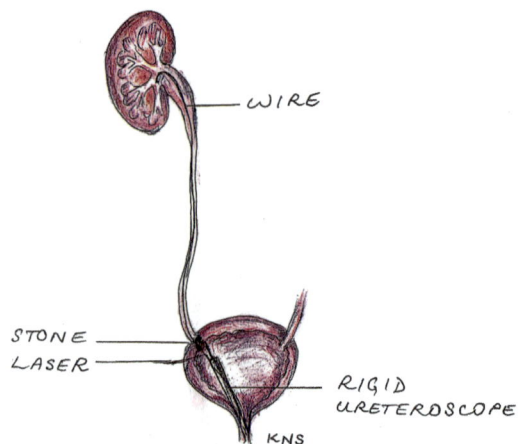

18.4   Patient Information and Consent-What to Tell the Patient

Why is this procedure being done?

- This procedure is being done to remove stones from the lower part of the ureter using a camera through the bladder
- Stones are broken up using a laser
- This procedure is done with cameras to avoid more major operations such as open surgery for stone removal
- A stent will be required at the end of the procedure, which may be removed in a few days (stent on strings) or a couple of weeks using a camera (Flexible cystoscope)
- The procedure is done as a daycase and followup will be in at a routine outpatient appointment

What are the alternatives

- Conservative management
- ESWL- shock wave therapy to the stone to try and break it up- may require 2 sessions, f this fails, usually surgery is required
- PCNL- using a camera through the back into the kidney, very large stones can be extracted
- Robotic or laparoscopic stone surgery- no commonly done for stones
- Open stone surgery- not common done for stones

What the procedure entails

- A general anaesthetic is used
- Antibiotics are given pre-procedure
- A camera is inserted and contrast studies are done
- A camera and laser will be passed to the kidney
- The stone will be broken to fragments or removed or dusted
- A stent will be passed up to the kidney that will be removed at a later date

The outcome

- Infection, sepsis, HDU/ ITU stay
- Bleeding
- Recurrence
- Remnant stone requiring further treatment
- Failure to reach stone requiring stenting and a 2nd look procedure or nephrostomy
- Trauma to the ureter- abrasion, stricture, mucosal damage, ureteric reconstruction
- Anaesthetic risks - MI, CVA, PE, DVT, Chest infection

18.5   Impact of ODE Inhibitors as Medical Expulsive Therapy on Ureteric Stones

Celik evaluated the effect of tadalafil compared with four alpha blockers (alfuzosin, doxazosin, tamsulosin and silodosin) as medical expulsive treatment for ureteral stones in male adults (Celik, 2018). Male adults who were admitted to urology clinic with flank pain and diagnosed with non complicated < 10 mm ureteral stone on non-contrast computed tomography (NCCT) between June 2014-September 2015 were retrospectively evaluated (Celik, 2018).

A total of 273 patients with ureteral stone were divided into five groups. Alfuzosin 10 mg/daily, doxazosin 8 mg/daily, tamsulosin 0.4 mg/daily, silodosin 8 mg/daily and tadalafil 5 mg/daily for 6 weeks were prescribed respectively (Celik, 2018). Age was higher in tadalafil group in distal stones (p = 0.032). Expulsion rate was found 78.1% for alfuzosin, 75.7% for doxazosin, 76.5% for tamsulosin, 88.6% for silodosin and 90% for tadalafil in distal (p = 0.44) and 21.7%, 30%, 30%, 30% and 54.5% in mid-proximal stones (p = 0.034) respectively (Celik, 2018).

Expulsion rate was higher in silodosin and tadalafil for distal ureteral stones but the difference didn't meet statistical significance (Celik, 2018). However the expulsion rate was significantly higher in tadalafil than in the other groups for mid-proximal ureteral stones (Celik, 2018). The result of this study showed that tadalafil may increases ureteric stone expulsion.

References

Akdeniz SÇF, Yildirim MA, Bozkurt O, Bulut MG, Hacihasanoglu ML, Demir O. Tadalafil versus alpha blockers (alfuzosin, doxazosin, tamsulosin and silodosin) as medical expulsive therapy for < 10 mm distal and proximal ureteral stones. Arch Ital Urol Androl. 2018;90(2):117–22.

NICE Guideline – Renal and Ureteric Stones: Assessment and Management: NICE. Renal and ureteric stones: assessment and management. BJU Int. 2019;123(2):220–32.

Pickard R, Starr K, MacLennan G, Kilonzo M, Lam T, Thomas R, Burr J, Norrie J, McPherson G, McDonald A, Shearer K, Gillies K, Boachie KAC, N'Dow J, Burgess N, Cameron TCS, McClinton S. Use of drug therapy in the management of symptomatic ureteric stones in hospitalised adults: a multicentre, placebo-controlled, randomised controlled trial and cost-effectiveness analysis of a calcium channel blocker (nifedipine) and an alpha-blocker (tamsulosin) (the SUSPEND trial). Health Technol Assess. 2015;19(63):vii–viii. 1–171

Surgical Strategy for Distal Ureteric Stones

19.1 Guidelines for Distal Ureteric Stones

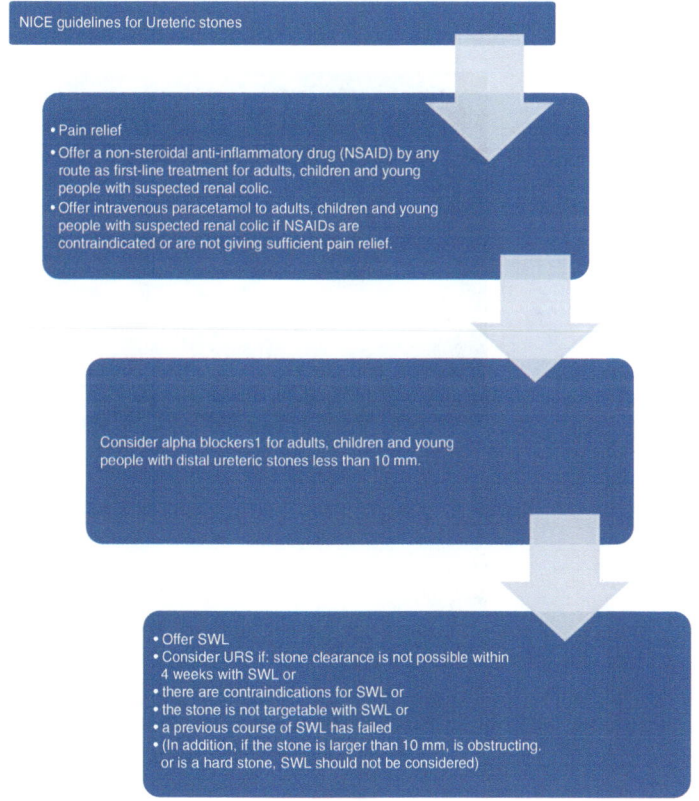

NICE guidelines for Ureteric stones

- Pain relief
- Offer a non-steroidal anti-inflammatory drug (NSAID) by any route as first-line treatment for adults, children and young people with suspected renal colic.
- Offer intravenous paracetamol to adults, children and young people with suspected renal colic if NSAIDs are contraindicated or are not giving sufficient pain relief.

Consider alpha blockers1 for adults, children and young people with distal ureteric stones less than 10 mm.

- Offer SWL
- Consider URS if: stone clearance is not possible within 4 weeks with SWL or
- there are contraindications for SWL or
- the stone is not targetable with SWL or
- a previous course of SWL has failed
- (In addition, if the stone is larger than 10 mm, is obstructing. or is a hard stone, SWL should not be considered)

NICE Guidelines, 2019

© The Author(s), under exclusive license to Springer Nature Switzerland AG 2021
S. S. Goonewardene et al., *Surgical Strategies in Endourology for Stone Disease*,
https://doi.org/10.1007/978-3-030-82143-2_19

19.2 Case 1

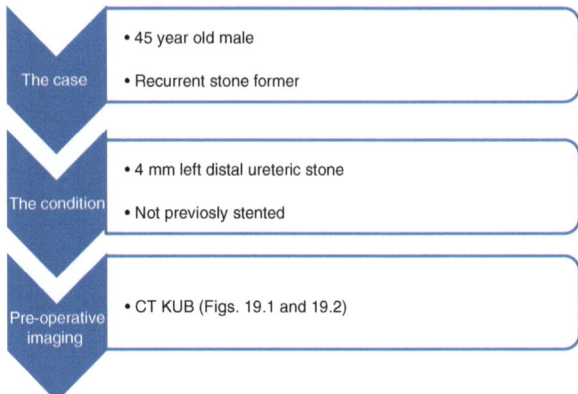

The case
• 45 year old male
• Recurrent stone former

The condition
• 4 mm left distal ureteric stone
• Not previosly stented

Pre-operative imaging
• CT KUB (Figs. 19.1 and 19.2)

Fig. 19.1 CT KUB

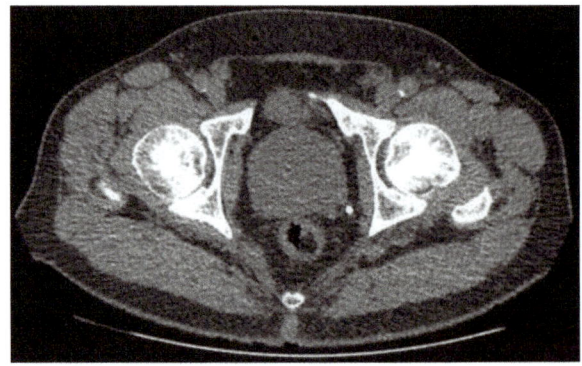

Fig. 19.2 CT KUB done
pre operative

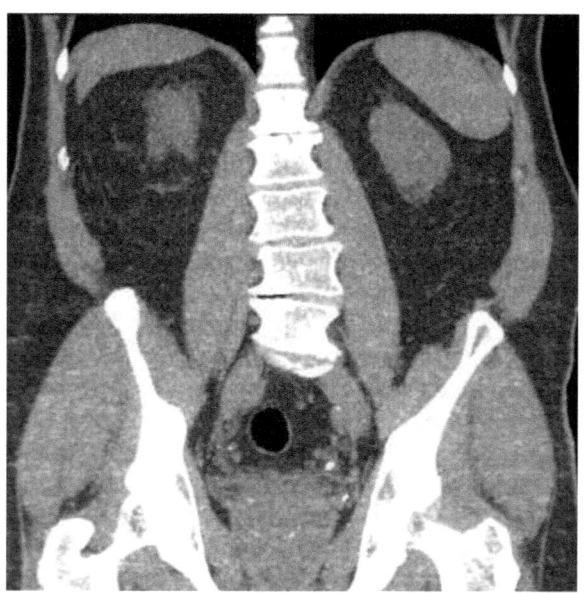

The equipment

- Sensor wire 0.08 -Frnitinol core over a hydrophilic coating
- Ureteric catheter white (soft) or blue (stiffer)
- Contrast-Urograffin 150 or 300.
- Long rigid ureteroscope
- Zero tip basket (tipless basket)
- Flexible ureteroscope, Access sheath on standby

The strategy

- Rigid cystoscope in, with bridge
- Pass sensor to renal pelvis
- Do a retrograde and identifiy distal ureteric stone
- Remove rigid cystoscope and ureteric catheter
- Using the long rigid, place the zero tip basket behind the stone
- Clear using the 265 laser fibre.
- Fragment and extract, start at 0.4/10 on laser settings (play it like a scale of music, if the stone is hard, increase the power).
- 6x24 fr stent

The difficulties

- The stone can often fly to the kidney- use a zero-tip basket to hold the stone and laser.
- It may be impacted into the wall lasering will be difficult, often resulting in stricture later and MAG 3 renogram to look for obstruction.
- The ureter may be tigh-you may have to stent and bring backt

The outcome

- Stones fully cleared from kidney.
- Chase stone type, then give diet advice accordingly.
- Stent register tract stent and ensure it is removed.
- Dietary advice including BAUS information leaflet.
- TFTs, Calcium, Urate , PTH.

19.3   Distal Ureteric Stones and Tamsulosin

Distal ureteric stones and tamsulosin

Furyk conducted a randomized, double-blind, placebocontrolled, multicentre trial . Patients were allocated to 0.4 mg of tamsulosin or placebo daily for 28 days. The primary outcomes were stone expulsion on CT at 28 days and time to stone expulsion. (Furyk, 2016)

There were 403 patients randomized. Stone passage occurred in 140 of 161 (87.0%) in the tamsulosin group and 127 of 155 (81.9%) with placebo, a difference of 5.0% (95% confidence interval -3.0% to 13.0%).

There was no difference in urologic interventions, time to self-reported stone passage, pain, or analgesia requirements. Adverse events were generally mild and did not differ between groups (Furyk, 2016).

There was no difference in either group in terms of spontaneous passage, time to stone passage, pain, or analgesia requirements.

In the subgroup with large stones (5 to 10 mm), tamsulosin did increase passage and should be considered. (Furyk, 2016)

19.4   Case 2

| The case | • 65 year old male
• Incidental finding of ureteric stone |

| The condition | • 7 mm right distal ureteric stone
• Not pre-stented |

| Pre-operative imaging | • CT KUB (Figs. 19.3 and 19.4) |

Fig. 19.3 CT scan
demonstrating right distal
ureteric stone

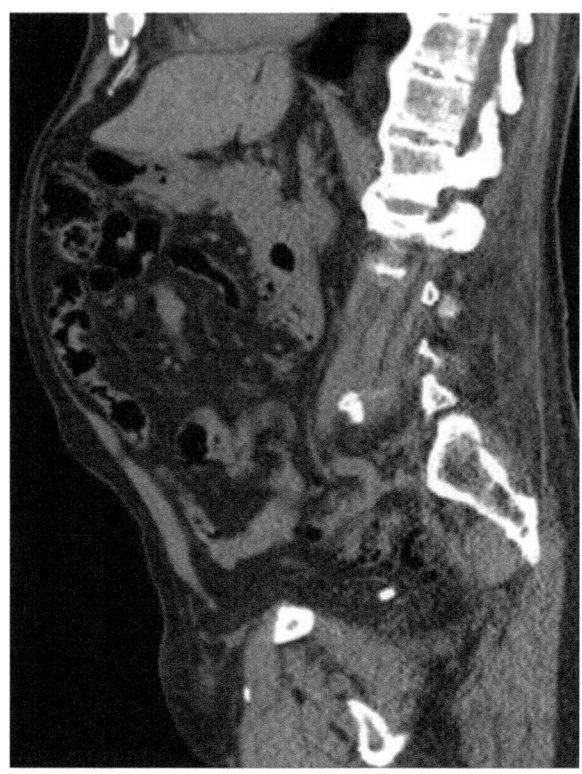

Fig. 19.4 CT
demonstrating 7 mm right
distal ureteric stone

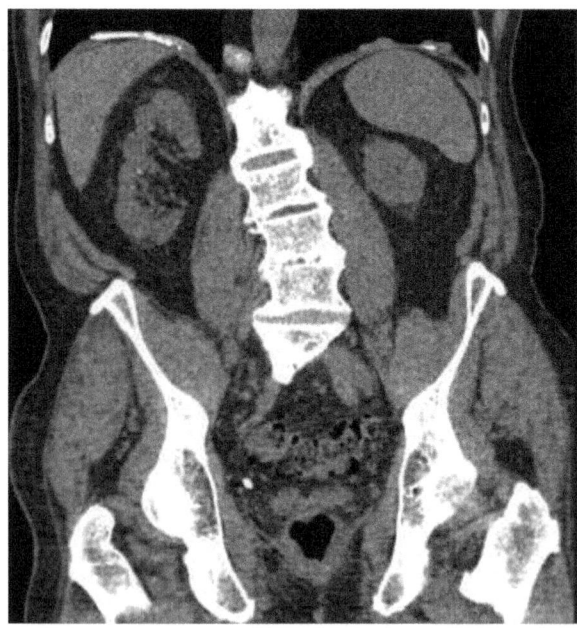

The equipment

- Sensor wire 0.08 Fr- nitinol core over a hydrophilic coating
- Ureteric catheter- white (soft) or blue (stiffer)
- Contrast- Urograffin 150 or 300.
- Long rigid ureteroscope
- Zero tip basket (tipless basket)
- Flexible ureteroscope, Access sheath on standby
  The strategy

The strategy

- Rigid cystoscope in, with bridge
- Pass sensor to renal pelvis
- Do a retrograde and identifiy distal ureteric stone
- Remove rigid cystoscope and ureteric catheter
- Using the long rigid, place the zero tip basket behind the stone
- Clear using the 265 laser fibre.
- Fragment and extract, start at 0.4/10 on laser settings (play it like a scale of music, if the stone is hard, increase the power).
- 6x24 fr stent

The difficulties

- The stone can often fly to the kidney- use a zero-tip basket to hold the stone and laser.
- It may be impacted into the wall- lasering will be difficult, often resulting in stricture later and MAG 3 renogram to look for obstruction.
- The ureter may be tight- you may have to stent and bring back
- You may not be able to reach the stone- a stent may be required, to simply open the ureter prior to a 2nd procedure.

The outcome

- Stones fully cleared from kidney.
- Chase stone type, then give diet advice accordingly.
- Stent register- tract stent and ensure it is removed.
- Dietary advice including BAUS information leaflet.
- Mag 3 renogram- to assess for stricture.
- TFTs, Calcium, Urate , PTH.

19.5   Case 3

- •55 year old male
- •Recurrent stone former

The case

- •5 mm left distal ureteric stone
- •Not previosly stented

The condition

- •CT KUB, Figs. 19.5 and 19.6

Pre-operative
imaging

Fig. 19.5 CT
demonstrating 5 mm distal
left ureteric stone

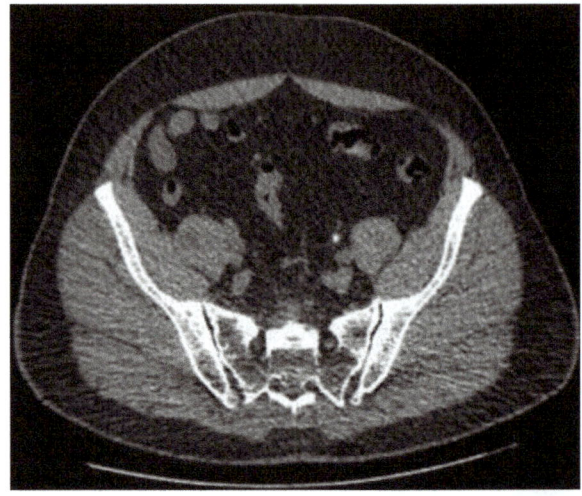

Fig. 19.6 CT
demonstrating 5 mm distal
left ureteric stone

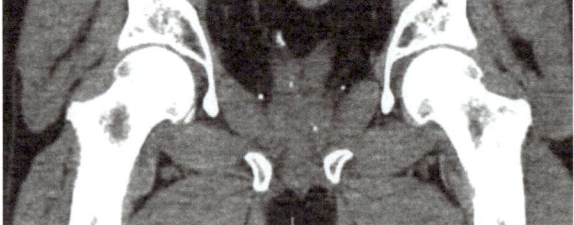

The equipment

- Sensor wire 0.08 Fr- nitinol core over a hydrophilic coating
- Ureteric catheter- white (soft) or blue (stiffer)
- Contrast- Urograffin 150 or 300.
- Long rigid ureteroscope
- Zero tip basket (tipless basket)
- Flexible ureteroscope, Access sheath on standby

The strategy

- Rigid cystoscope in, with bridge
- Pass sensor to renal pelvis
- Do a retrograde and identifiy distal ureteric stone
- Remove rigid cystoscope and ureteric catheter
- Using the long rigid, place the zero tip basket behind the stone
- Clear using the 265 laser fibre.
- Fragment and extract, start at 0.4/10 on laser settings (play it like a scale of music, if the stone is hard, increase the power).
- 6x24 fr stent

The difficulties

- The stone can often fly to the kidney- use a zero-tip basket to hold the stone and laser.
- It may be impacted into the wall- lasering will be difficult, often resulting in stricture later and MAG 3 renogram to look for obstruction.
- The ureter may be tight- you may have to stent and bring back
- You may not be able to reach the stone- a stent may be required, to simply open the ureter prior to a 2nd procedure.

The outcome

- Stones fully cleared from kidney.
- Chase stone type, then give diet advice accordingly.
- Stent register- tract stent and ensure it is removed.
- Dietary advice including BAUS information leaflet.
- Mag 3 renogram- to assess for stricture.
- TFTs, Calcium, Urate , PTH.

19.6   Case 4

The case
- 65 year old male
- Recurrent stone former

The condition
- Incidental Finding 9mm Right Distal ureteric Calculus at different hospital
- Fit paitient

Pre-operative imaging
- CT KUB (Figs. 19.7, 19.8, 19.9 and 19.10)

Fig. 19.7 CT KUB demonstrating 7 mm right distal ureteric stone

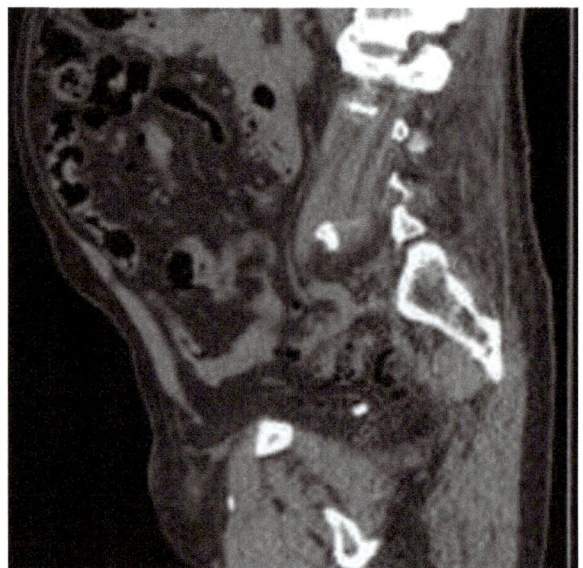

Fig. 19.8 CT KUB
demonstrating right distal
ureteric stone

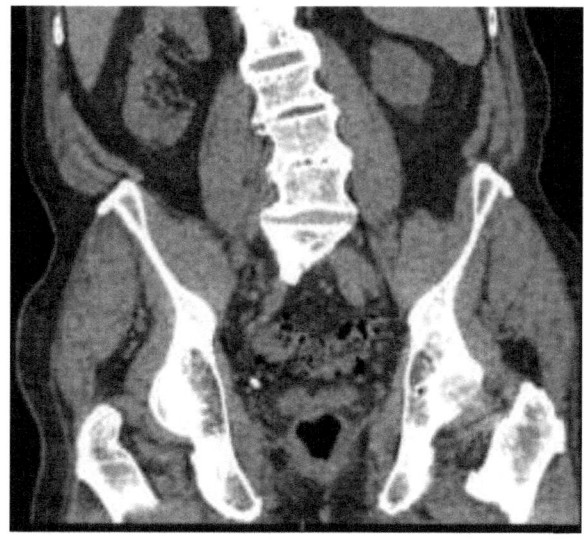

Fig. 19.9 Retrograde
done at time of emergency
stenting identifying stone

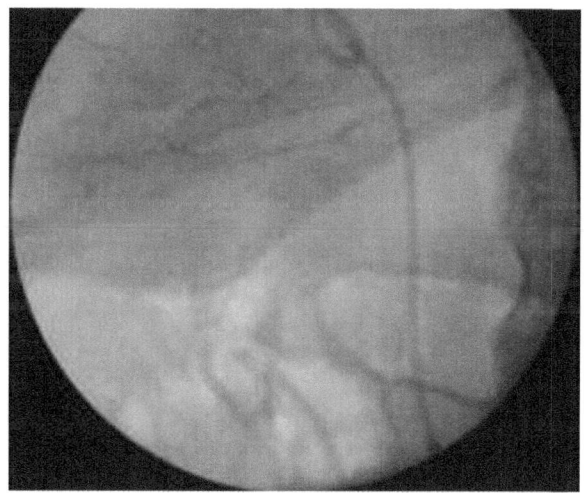

Fig. 19.10 Demonstrating
management of a distal
ureteric stone

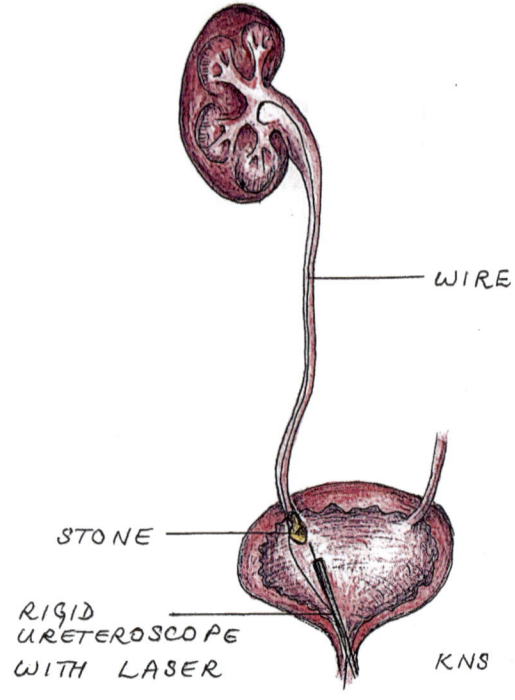

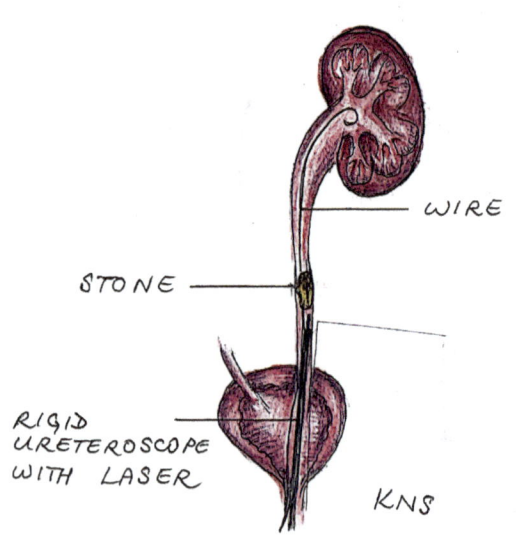

The equipment

- Sensor wire 0.08 Fr- nitinol core over a hydrophilic coating
- Ureteric catheter- white (soft) or blue (stiffer)
- Contrast- Urograffin 150 or 300.
- Long rigid ureteroscope
- Zero tip basket (tipless basket)
- FLexible ureteroscope, Access sheath on standby

The strategy

- Rigid cystoscope in, with bridge
- Pass sensor to renal pelvis
- Do a retrograde and identifiy distal ureteric stone
- Remove rigid cystoscope and ureteric catheter
- Using the long rigid, place the zero tip basket behind the stone
  (sometimes, the ureter is too tight, you may not be able to do this).
- Clear using the 265 laser fibre.
- Fragment and extract, start at 0.4/10 on laser settings (play it like a
  scale of music, if the stone is hard, increase the power).
- 6x24 fr stent

The difficulties

- The stone can often fly to the kidney- use a zero-tip basket to hold the
  stone and laser.
- It may be impacted into the wall- lasering will be difficult, often resulting in
  stricture later and MAG 3 renogram to look for obstruction.
- The ureter may be tight- you may have to stent and bring back
- Do not push or force the ureteroscope-- it has a sharp tip, you do not want
  to end up outside the ureter.

The outcome

- Stones fully cleared from kidney.
- Chase stone type, then give diet advice accordingly.
- Stent register- tract stent and ensure it is removed.
- Dietary advice including BAUS information leaflet.
- TFTs, Calcium, Urate , PTH.

19.7   Case 4

The case
- 45 year old male

=The condition
- 5 mm left distal ureteric stone
- Prior emergency stent, size unknown

Pre-operative imaging
- CT KUB
- Pyelogram (Figs. 19.11, 19.12 and 19.13)

Fig. 19.11 CT demonstrating distal ureteric stone

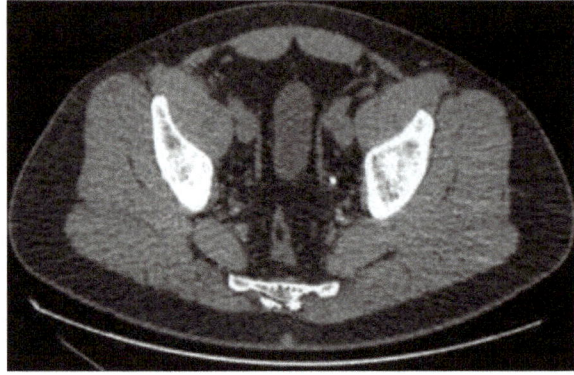

Fig. 19.12 CT
demonstrating distal
ureteric stone

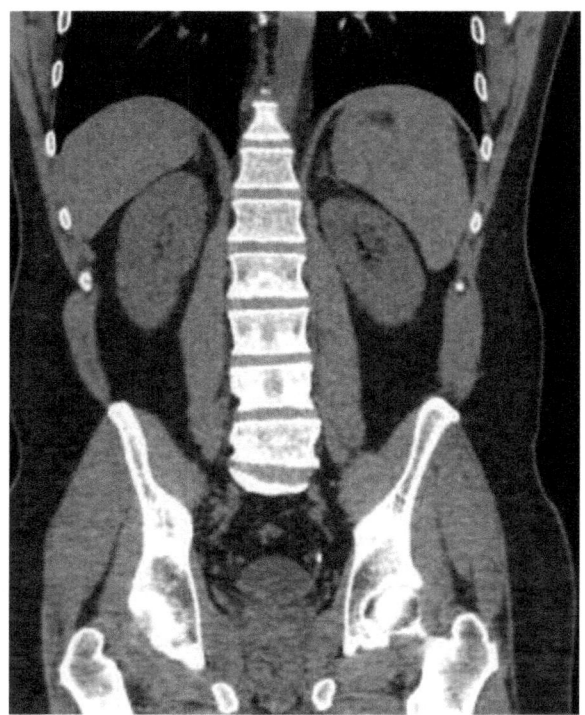

Fig. 19.13 Stone on
fluoroscopy at emergency
stenting

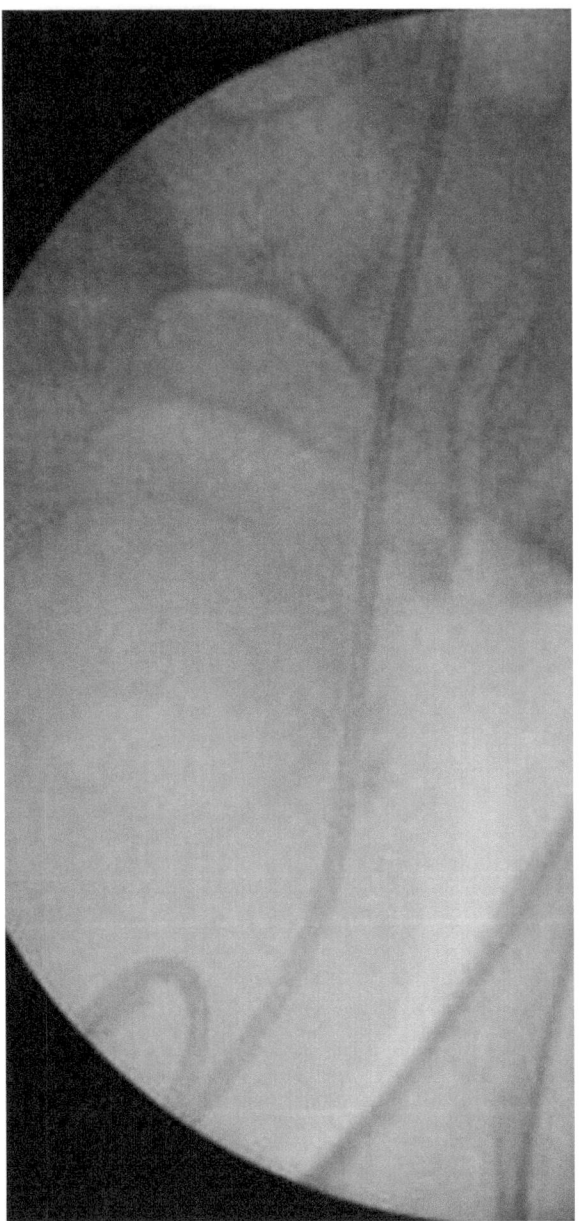

The equipment

- Sensor wire 0.08 Fr- nitinol core over a hydrophilic coating
- Ureteric catheter- white (soft) or blue (stiffer)
- Contrast- Urograffin 150 or 300.
- Long rigid ureteroscope
- Zero tip basket (tipless basket)
- Flexible ureteroscope
- Access sheath on standby

The strategy

- Rigid cystoscope in, with bridge
- Pass sensor to renal pelvis
- Remove stent with biopsy forceps
- Do a retrograde and identifiy distal ureteric stone
- Remove rigid cystoscope and ureteric catheter
- Using the long rigid, place the zero tip basket behind the stone
- Clear using the 265 laser fibre.
- Fragment and extract, start at 0.4/10 on laser settings (play it like a scale of music, if the stone is hard, increase the power).
- 6x24 fr stent

The difficulties

- The stone can often fly to the kidney- use a zero-tip basket to hold the stone and laser.
- It may be impacted into the wall- lasering will be difficult, often resulting in stricture later and MAG 3 renogram to look for obstruction.
- The ureter may be tight- you may have to stent and bring back
- It may have passed- always make sure these patients have an upto date CT.

The outcome

- Stones fully cleared from kidney.
- Chase stone type, then give diet advice accordingly.
- Stent register- tract stent and ensure it is removed.
- Dietary advice including BAUS information leaflet.
- TFTs, Calcium, Urate , PTH.

19.8   Patient Information and Consent

Why is this procedure being done?

- This procedure is being done to remove stones from the lower part of the tube from the kidney to the bladder
- Thisv uses a camera through the bladder
- Stones are broken up using a laser
- This procedure is done with cameras to avoid more major operations such as open surgery for stone removal
- A stent will be required at the end of the procedure, which may be removed in a few days (stent on strings) or a couple of weeks using a camera (Flexible cystoscope)
- The procedure is done as a daycase and followup will be in at a routine outpatient appointment

What are the alternatives

- Conservative management
- ESWL- shock wave therapy to the stone to try and break it up- may require 2 sessions, f this fails, usually surgery is required
- PCNL- using a camera through the back into the kidney, very large stones can be extracted
- Robotic or laparoscopic stone surgery- no commonly done for stones
- Open stone surgery- not commonly done for stones

What the procedure entails

- A general anaesthetic is used
- Antibiotics are given pre-procedure
- A camera is inserted and studies are done
- A camera and laser will be passed to the kidney
- The stone will be broken to fragments or removed or dusted
- A stent will be passed up to the kidney that will be removed at a later date

The outcome

- Infection, sepsis, HDU/ ITU stay
- Bleeding
- Recurrence
- Remnant stone requiring further treatment
- Failure to reach stone requiring stenting and a 2nd look procedure or nephrostomy
- Trauma to the ureter- abrasion, stricture, mucosal damage, ureteric reconstruction
- Anaesthetic risks - MI, CVA, PE, DVT, Chest infection

19.9   Surgical Strategy for a Difficult Distal Ureteric Stone

NICE guidelines for ureteric stones

- Pain relief
- Offer a non-steroidal anti-inflammatory drug (NSAID) by any route as first-line treatment for adults, children and young people with suspected renal colic.
- Offer intravenous paracetamol to adults, children and young people with suspected renal colic if NSAIDs are contraindicated or are not giving sufficient pain relief.

Consider alpha blockers for adults, children and young people with distal ureteric stones less than 10 mm (whilst this is in the guidance, from a practical point of view, an 8-10mm stone is unlikely to pass alone, requiring stenting or if available, primary ureteroscopy.

- Offer SWL
- Consider URS if: stone clearance is not possible within 4 weeks with SWL or
- There are contraindications for SWL or
- The stone is not targetable with SWL or
- A previous course of SWL has failed

19.10 Case 1

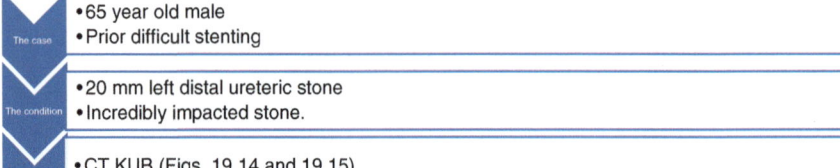

The case
- •65 year old male
- •Prior difficult stenting

The condition
- •20 mm left distal ureteric stone
- •Incredibly impacted stone.

Pre-operative imaging
- •CT KUB (Figs. 19.14 and 19.15)

Fig. 19.14 CT
Demonstrating 2 cm stone
in left distal ureter

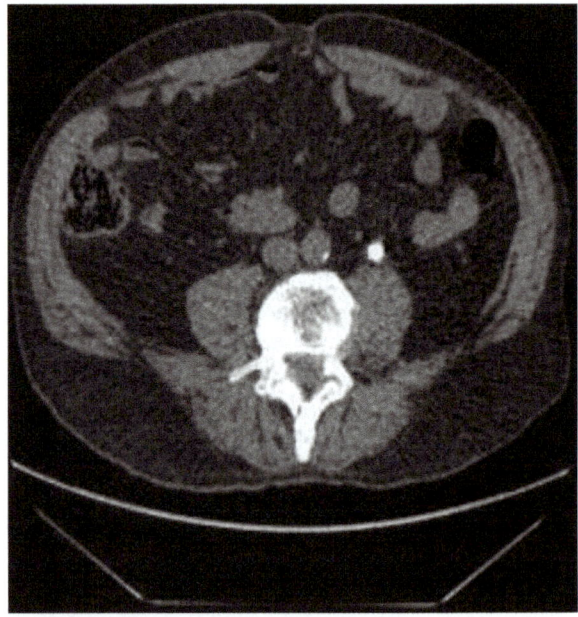

Fig. 19.15 CT
Demonstrating 2 cm stone
in left distal ureter

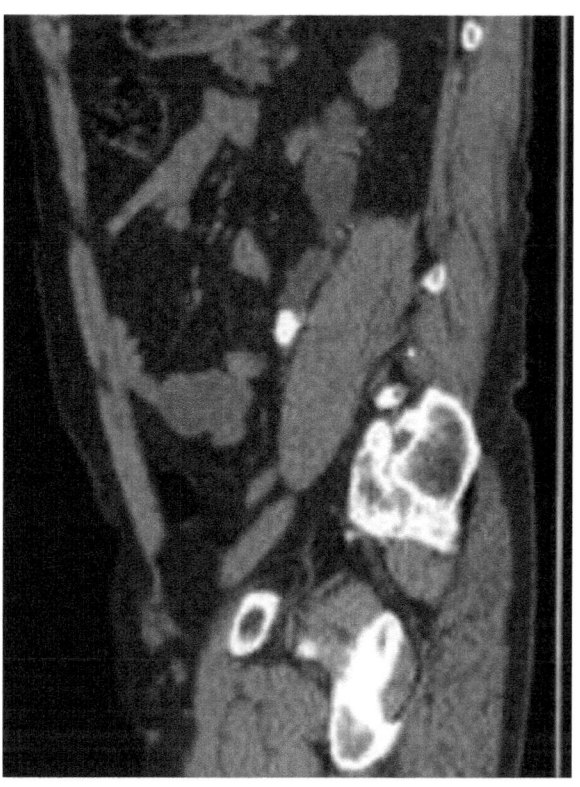

The equipment

- Sensor wire 0.08 Fr- nitinol core over a hydrophilic coating
- Ureteric catheter- white (soft) or blue (stiffer)
- Contrast- Urograffin 150 or 300.
- Long rigid ureteroscope
- Zero tip basket (tipless basket)
- Flexible ureteroscope, Access sheath on standby

The strategy

- Rigid cystoscope in, with bridge
- Pass sensor to renal pelvis - coil and clip
- Do a retrograde and identifiy distal ureteric stone
- Remove rigid cystoscope and ureteric catheter
- Using the long rigid, go up to stone,
- Clear using the 265 laser fibre.
- Aim to dust starting at at 0.4/10 on laser settings (play it like a scale of music, if the stone is hard, increase the power).
- 6x24 fr stent

The difficulties

- Passing the guidewire past the stone- it was a difficult initial emergency stenting.
- The stone was significantly impacted into the wall- lasering will be difficult, often resulting in stricture later and MAG 3 renogram to look for obstruction.
- The ureter may be tight- you may have to stent and bring back
- Aim to dust- the vision will often be poor.

The outcome

- Stone fully cleared from kidney.
- Chase stone type, then give diet advice accordingly.
- Stent register- track the stent and ensure it is removed.
- Mag 3 renogram at 3 months post stent removal.
- Dietary advice including BAUS information leaflet.
- TFTs, Calcium, Urate , PTH.

19.11 Patient Information and Consent: What to Tell Patients

Why is this procedure being done?
- This procedure is being done to remove stones from the lower part of the ureter using a camera through the bladder
- Stones are broken up using a laser
- This procedure is done with cameras to avoid more major operations such as open surgery for stone removal
- A stent will be required at the end of the procedure, which may be removed in a few days (stent on strings) or a couple of weeks using a camera (Flexible cystoscope)
- The procedure is done as a daycase and followup will be in at a routine outpatient appointment

What are the alternatives
- Conservative management
- ESWL- shock wave therapy to the stone to try and break it up- may require 2 sessions, f this fails, usually surgery is required
- Robotic or laparoscopic stone surgery- no commonly done for stones
- Open stone surgery - not commonly done for stones

What the procedure entails
- A general anaesthetic is used
- Antibiotics are given pre-procedure
- A camera is inserted and constrast studies are done
- A camera and laser will be passed to the kidney
- The stone will be broken to fragments or removed or dusted
- A stent will be passed up to the kidney that will be removed at a later date

The outcome
- Infection, sepsis, HDU/ ITU stay
- Bleeding
- Recurrence
- Remnant stone requiring further treatment
- Failure to reach stone requiring stenting and a 2nd look procedure or nephrostomy
- Trauma to the ureter- abrasion, stricture, mucosal damage, ureteric reconstruction
- Anaesthetic risks - MI, CVA, PE, DVT, Chest infection

References

Furyk JS, Chu K, Banks C, Greenslade J, Keijzers G, Thom O, Torpie T, Dux C, Narula R. Distal ureteric stones and tamsulosin: a double-blind, placebo-controlled, randomized, multicenter trial. Ann Emerg Med. 2016;67(1):86–95.e2.

NICE Guideline – Renal and Ureteric Stones: Assessment and Management: NICE. Renal and ureteric stones: assessment and management. BJU Int. 2019;123(2):220–32.

Turk C, Petrik A, Sarica K, Seitz C, Skolarikos A, Straub M, Knoll T. EAU guidelines on diagnosis and conservative management of urolithiasis. Eur Urol. 2016a;69(3):468–74.

Turk C, Petrik A, Sarica K, Seitz C, Skolarikos A, Straub M, Knoll T. EAU guidelines on interventional treatment for urolithiasis. Eur Urol. 2016b;69(3):475–82.

Surgical Strategy for Stones Within a Calyceal Diverticula

20

20.1   Calyceal Diverticular, Indications for Management

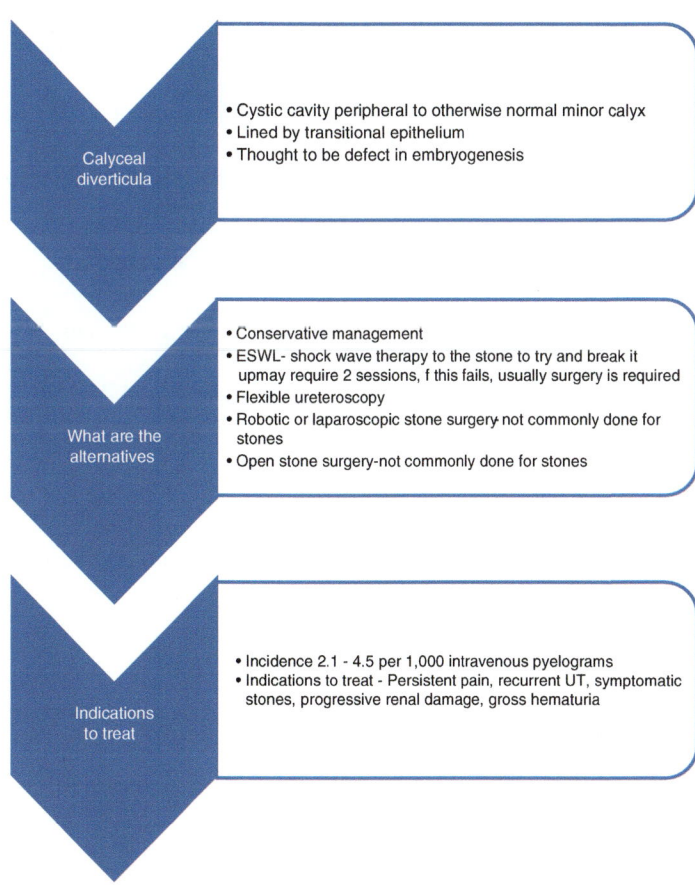

Calyceal diverticula
- Cystic cavity peripheral to otherwise normal minor calyx
- Lined by transitional epithelium
- Thought to be defect in embryogenesis

What are the alternatives
- Conservative management
- ESWL- shock wave therapy to the stone to try and break it upmay require 2 sessions, f this fails, usually surgery is required
- Flexible ureteroscopy
- Robotic or laparoscopic stone surgery- not commonly done for stones
- Open stone surgery-not commonly done for stones

Indications to treat
- Incidence 2.1 - 4.5 per 1,000 intravenous pyelograms
- Indications to treat - Persistent pain, recurrent UT, symptomatic stones, progressive renal damage, gross hematuria

© The Author(s), under exclusive license to Springer Nature
Switzerland AG 2021
S. S. Goonewardene et al., *Surgical Strategies in Endourology for Stone Disease*,
https://doi.org/10.1007/978-3-030-82143-2_20

20.2   Role of PCNL in Calyceal Diverticular Stones

Calyceal diverticula are rare entities that can pose a significant challenge when it comes to their management (Smyth, 2019).

PCNL now plays a key part in the management of these stones (Smyth, 2019). The increasing accessibility of robotics has a role to play in the management of this condition but is not likely to surpass flexible ureteroscopic (fURS) or percutaneous approaches (Smyth, 2019).

The future of surgical management for this condition lies in striking a balance between treatment efficacy and invasiveness (Smyth, 2019).

20.3   Case 1: ESWL Then Flexible Ureterorenoscopy for a Calyceal Diverticula Stone

The case

- 60 year old female
- Pain intermittently in right flank
- Recurrent UTIS

The condition and indications to treat

- Two tiny stones in calyceal diverticula
- Two episodes of ESWL failed
- Patient is still getting pain and recurrent UTIS

Pre-operative imaging

- CT KUB
- Incidence of stones Cystic cavity peripheral to otherwise normal minor calyx
- Lined by transitional epithelium
- Thought to be defect in embryogenesis
- Incidence 2.1 - 4.5 per 1,000 intravenous pyelograms
- Middleton, 1974 10%
- Timmons, 1975 39%
- Williams, 1969 50%

Pre-op surgical strategy

- Rigid cystoscope in, with bridge (Figs. 20.1, 20.2, 20.3 and 20.4)
- Pass sensor to renal pelvis
- Do a retrograde to identify stone
- Using the long rigid, assess the ureter is clear 1st.
- Pass access sheath, 9/11 35 long in female, to renal pelvis under Xray screening
- Railroad flexi up to kidney.
- Identify diverticula and laser open neck.
- Fragment and extract, start at 0.4/ 10 on laser settings
- Extract using zero-tip basket
- 6x24 fr stent

Fig. 20.1 Stones within a calyceal diverticula

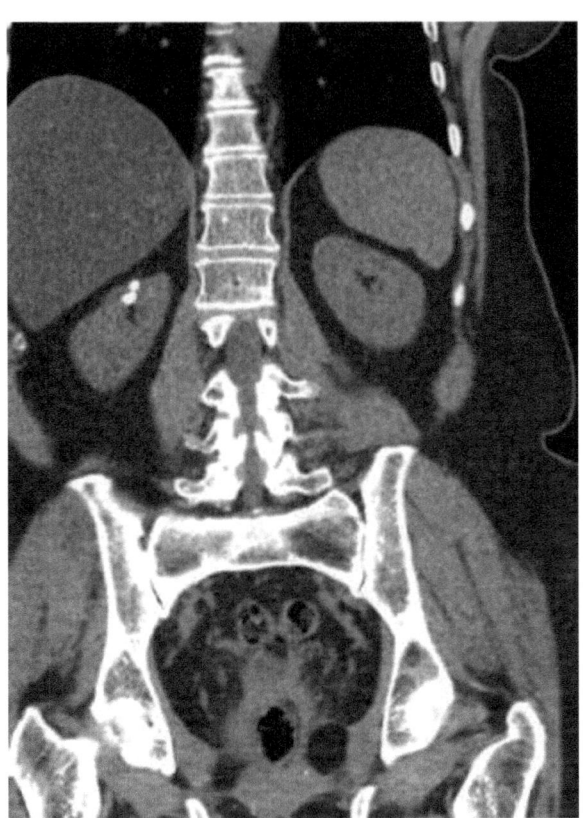

Fig. 20.2 Pyelogram demonstrating stones in calyceal diverticulum

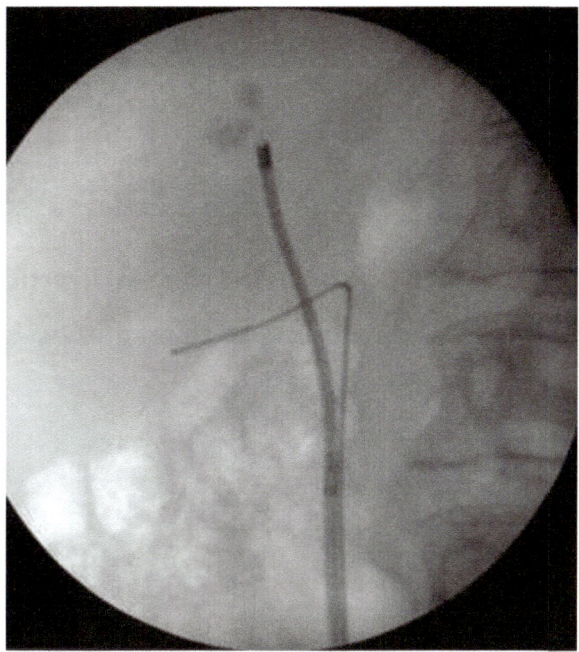

Fig. 20.3 Demonstrating access to a calyceal diverticula stone

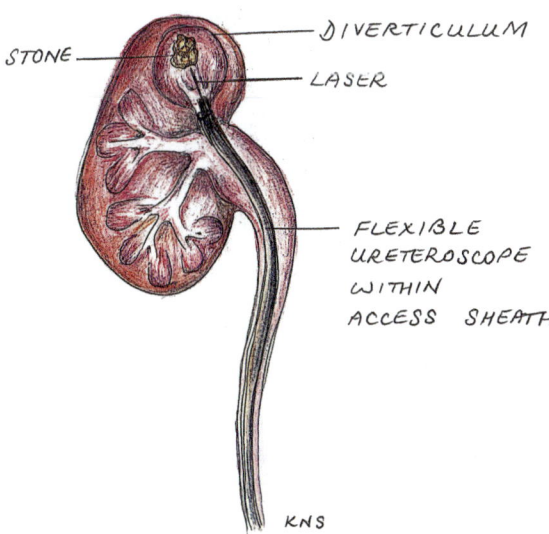

STONE

DIVERTICULUM

LASER

FLEXIBLE URETEROSCOPE WITHIN ACCESS SHEATH

KNS

Fig. 20.4   The Access
Sheath

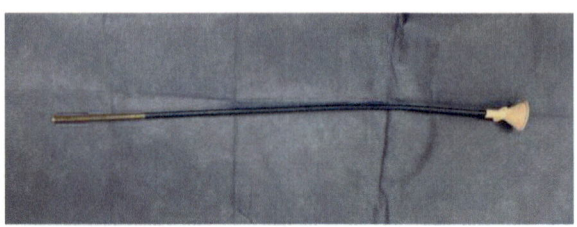

20.4   ESWL Outcomes in Calyceal Diverticular Stones

Fragmentation successful in all patients with
30% re-treatment rate
  Patients Residual Stones
  20%   None
  30%   > 50% remaining
  50%   < 50% remaining
70% of patients had resolution of symptoms
Psiharamis & Dretler, 1987

Relatively small (< 1.5 cm) calculi (n=19)
Radiographically patent diverticular neck
Initial stone-free rate   -   58%
Symptom-free rate   -   86%
Recurrent infection   -   67%
Streem & Yost, 1992

20.5   Case 2 Combination Therapy for a Calyceal Diverticular Stone

The case	• 45 year old male • Pilot

The conditio	• Two left upper pole stones • Likely in a calyceal diverticula • Combination approach of Flexible ureteroscopy +/- ESWL

Pre-operative imaging	• Xray KUB and IVU (Figs. 20.5 and 20.6)

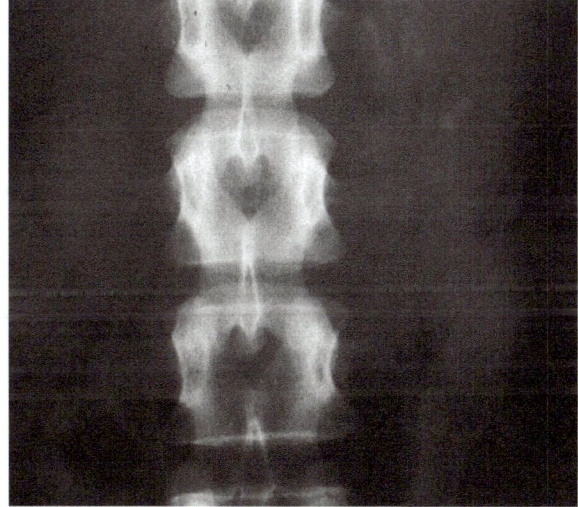

Fig. 20.5 Xray KUB—stones in a calyceal diverticula

Fig. 20.6 IVU

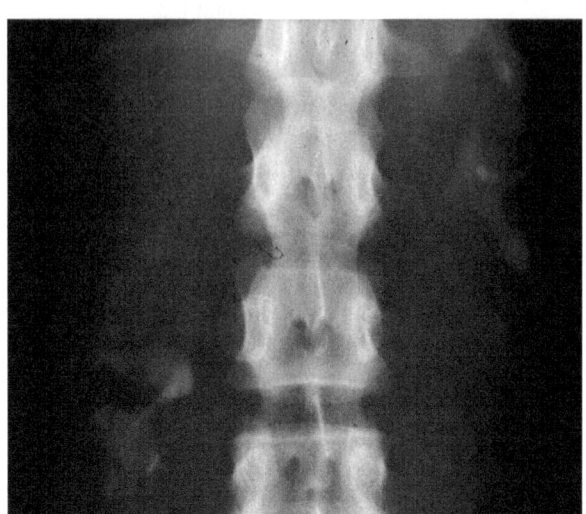

The equipment

- Sensor wire 0.08 Fr- nitinol core over a hydrophilic coating
- Ureteric catheter- white (soft) or blue (stiffer)
- Contrast- Urograffin 150 or 300.
- Long rigid ureteroscope
- Flexible ureteroscope
- Access sheath 9/11 35 fr- calibrate to ureteric size

The strategy

- During the procedure, the ureter was clear of stone
- There was no other stone in the kidney, except that in the calyceal diverticula
- The neck was lasered open.
- The stones were successfully fragmented and extracted
- A stent was placed at the end

The difficulties

- Finding the calyx- sometimes the neck is so narrow, you overshoot it
- Sometimes you can be looking straight at it and you shoot past it
- Lasering open the calyceal neck- it can be very tough
- Poor vision- go for fragmentation and extraction over dusting
- Very often, there is no neck at all- the stones are embedded in the renal parenchyma.

The outcome

- The diverticula neck was successfully lasered open, and stone free.
- The stent was removed post operatively
- Bloods were checked for Urate, Calcium
- As the stones were not in the collecting system, so no further follow up was needed

20.6   Outcomes from Calyceal Diverticular Stones

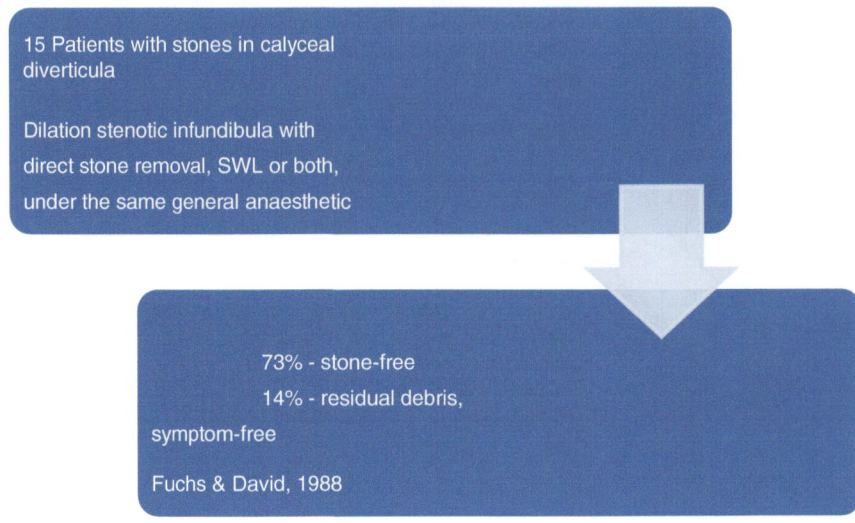

15 Patients with stones in calyceal diverticula

Dilation stenotic infundibula with
direct stone removal, SWL or both,
under the same general anaesthetic

73% - stone-free
14% - residual debris,
symptom-free
Fuchs & David, 1988

Please see Fig. 20.7 for Intraoperative imaging and placement of a safety wire.

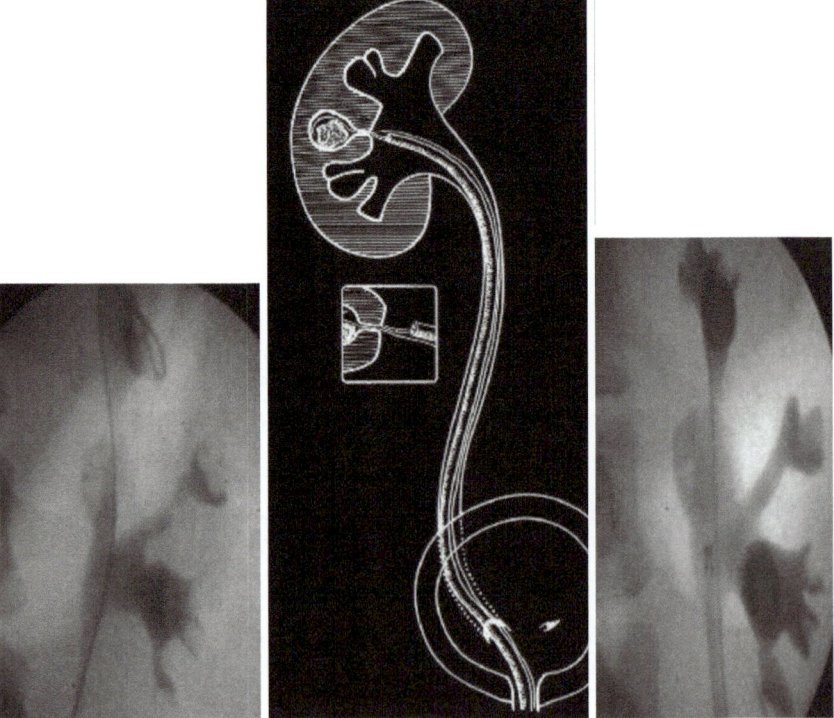

Fig. 20.7   Intraoperative imaging—placement of safety wire

20.7   Case 3 Role of PCNL Monotherapy with Calyceal Diverticular Stones

The case
- 65 year old female
- Primary presentation

The condition
- An 8 mm stone in a right upper pole calyceal diverticula

Pre-operative imaging
- Xray KUB and IVU (Figs. 20.8 and 20.9)

Fig. 20.8 Xray KUB from theatre

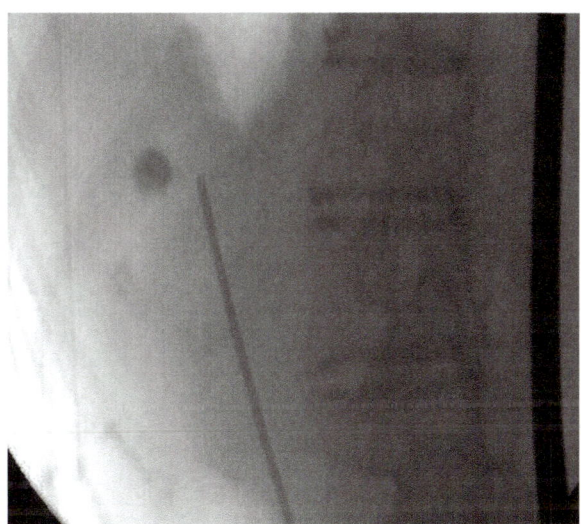

Fig. 20.9 Retrograde conducted in theatre

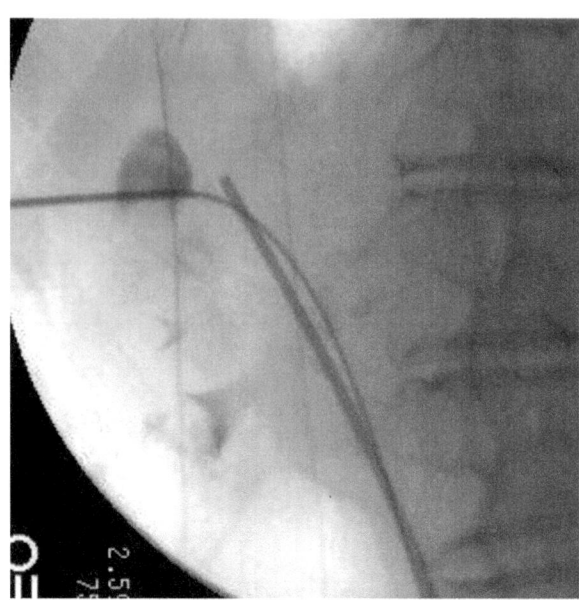

Fig. 20.10 Placement of needle for PCNL tract

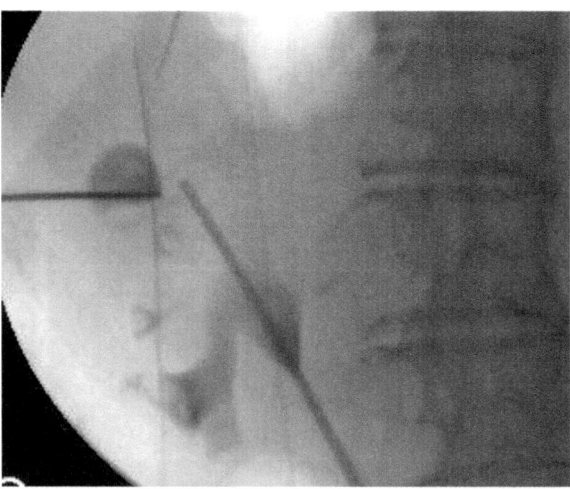

Fig. 20.11 Insertion of safety wire

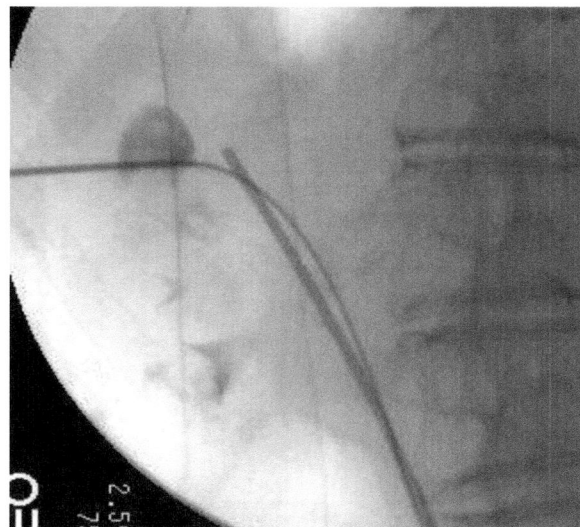

Fig. 20.12 Insertion of balloon dilator and dilation of tract

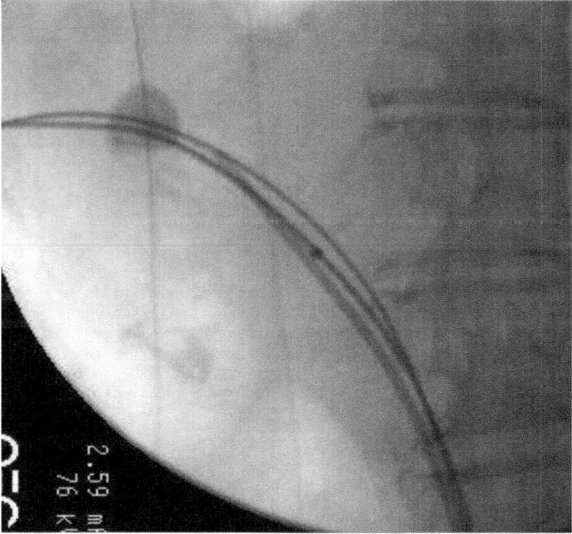

Fig. 20.13 Dilation of tract

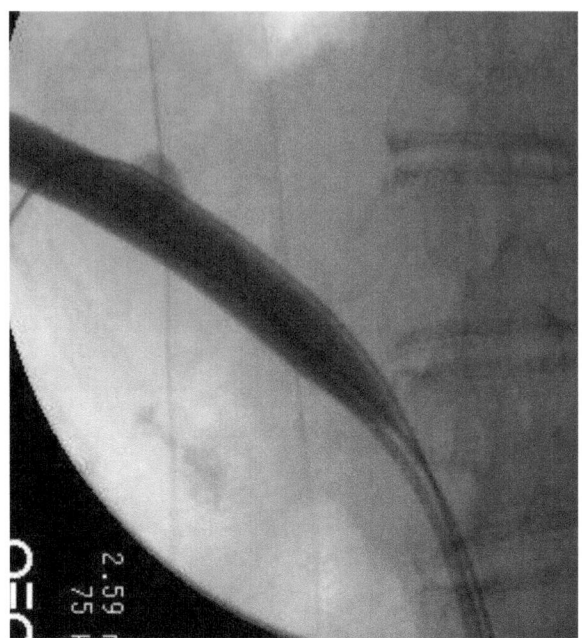

Fig. 20.14 Insertion of sheath

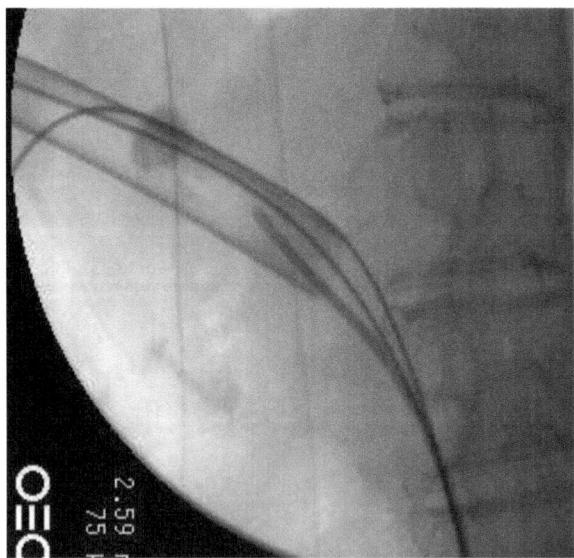

Fig. 20.15 Insertion of nephroscope

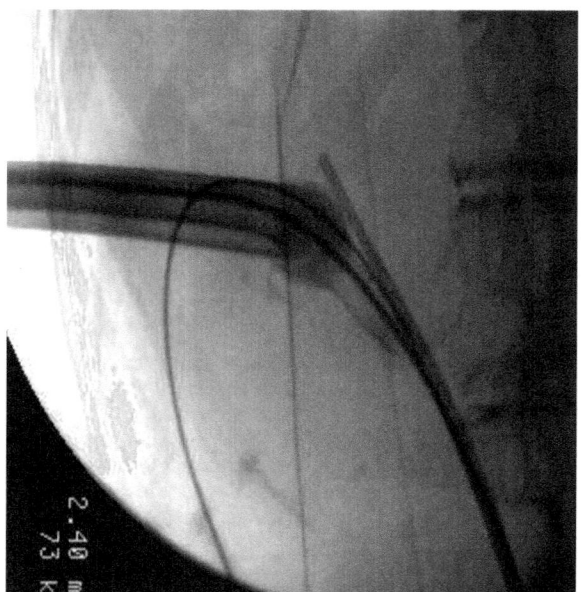

The equipment

- Sensor wire 0.08 Fr- nitinol core over a hydrophilic coating
- Ureteric balloon catheter
- Contrast- Urograffin 150 or 300.
- Rigid nephroscope
- Flexible nephroscope
- Ultrasonic device
- Pneumatic device
- Flexible ureteroscope

The strategy

- Rigid cystoscope in, with bridge
- Do cystoscopy and retrograde study
- Place ureteric balloon catheter
- Identify stones with fluoroscopy, or us
- Using seldinger technique, place tract and perc onto stone
- Using nephroscope fragment stone and extract
- Place nephrostomy and stent

The difficulties

- Piercing onto the stone without injuring adjacent viscera
- Properly clearing stone, which may require multiple punctures
- Rate of vascular injury is higher in lower pole stone compared to mid calyceal stone
- **Vascular injury through infundibulum puncture**
- **UC   - 67.6% (PSA)***
- **LC   - 68.2%**
- **MC   - 38.4%**
- *** PSA = Posterior Segmental Artery crossing (57%)**

The outcome

- Stones fully cleared from kidney.
- Chase stone type.
- Stent register- tract stent and ensure it is removed.
- Dietary advice including BAUS information leaflet.
- TFTs, Calcium, Urate .
- Figures 20.10, 20.11, 20.12, 20.13, 20.14 and 20.15

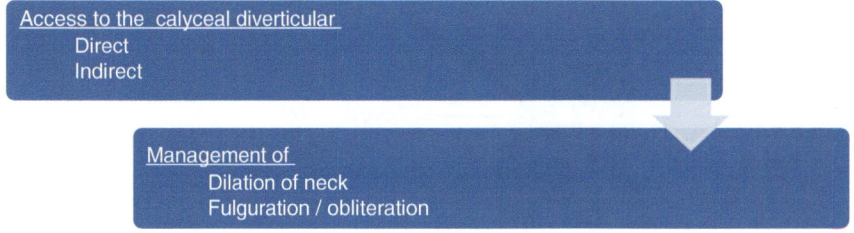

Access to the calyceal diverticular
    Direct
    Indirect

Management of
    Dilation of neck
    Fulguration / obliteration

20.8   Calyceal Access in Calyceal Diverticular Stones

Figures 20.16 and 20.17 Direct and indirect access to a calyceal stone

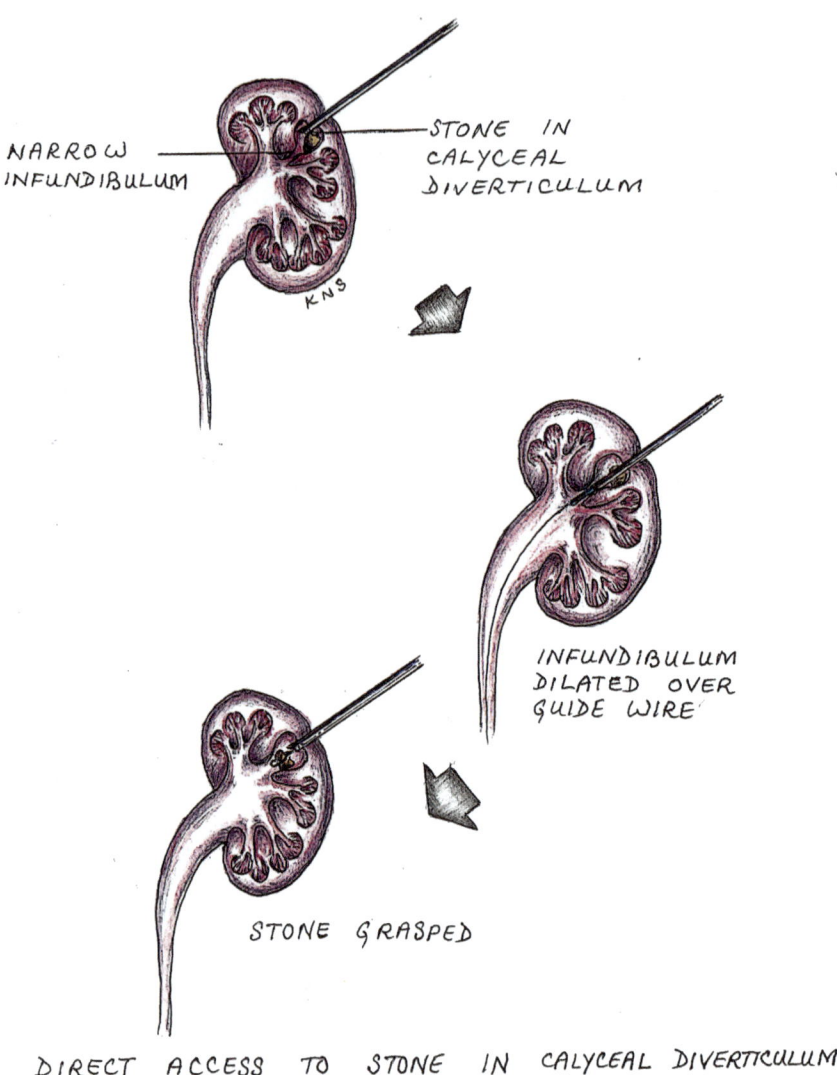

DIRECT ACCESS TO STONE IN CALYCEAL DIVERTICULUM

Fig. 20.16 Direct access to stone

Fig. 20.17 Indirect access to stone

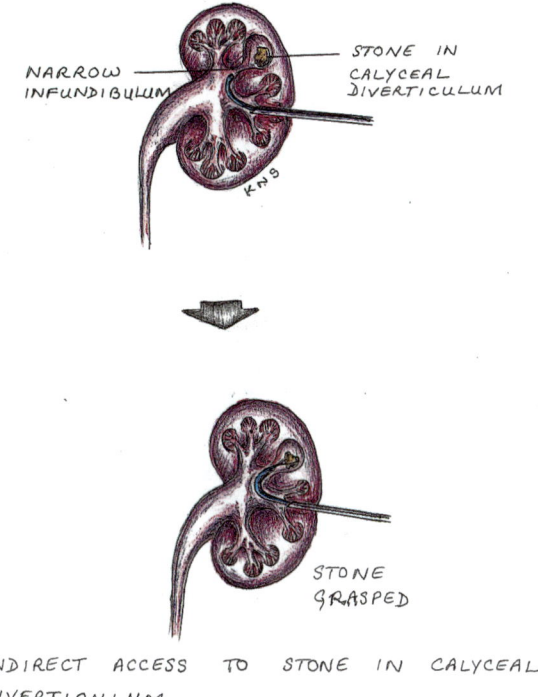

INDIRECT ACCESS TO STONE IN CALYCEAL DIVERTICULUM

20.9   Case 4 Ureteroscopic Access to a Calyceal Diverticular Stone

The case
- 45 year old male
- Chronic backache

The condition
- Multiple tiny right upper pole stones
- Within a calyceal diverticulum

Pre-operative imaging
- Xray KUB and IVU (Figs. 20.18, 20.19, 20.20, 20.21, 20.22, 20.23 and 20.24)

Fig. 20.18 Xray KUB

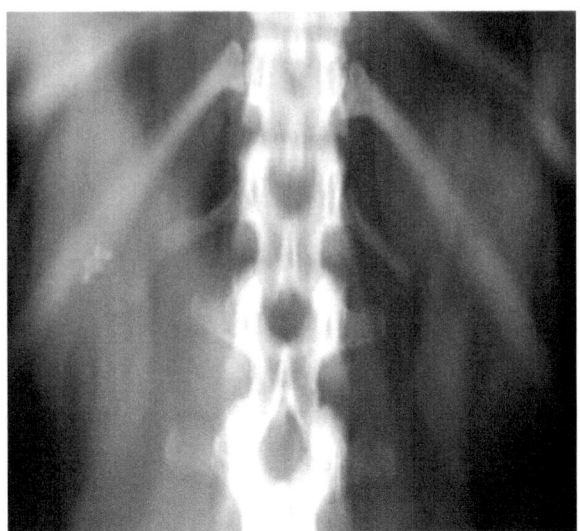

Fig. 20.19 Preop IVU

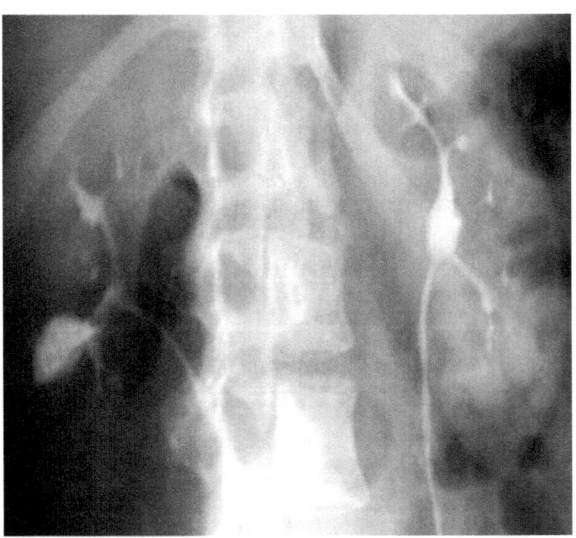

Fig. 20.20 Identification of the neck of the diverticulum

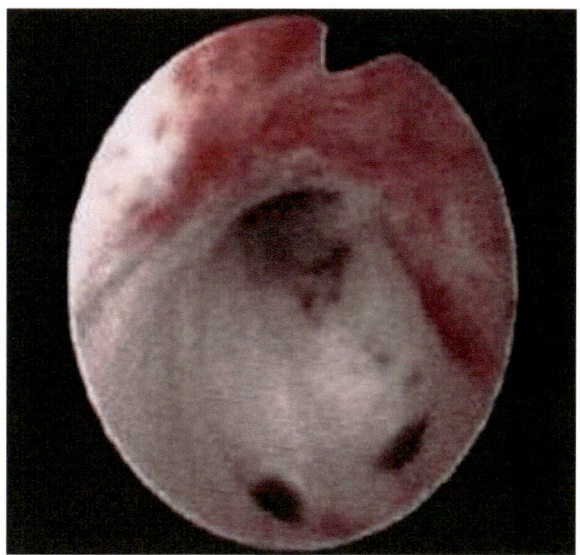

Fig. 20.21 Incision of the Infundibulum

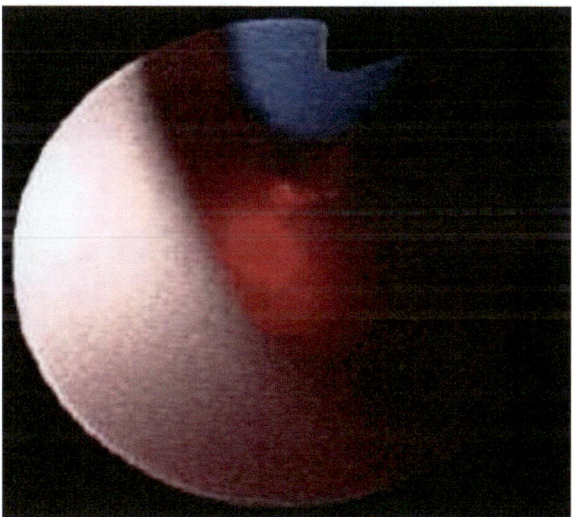

Fig. 20.22 Guidewire passed to diverticulum with scope railroaded up

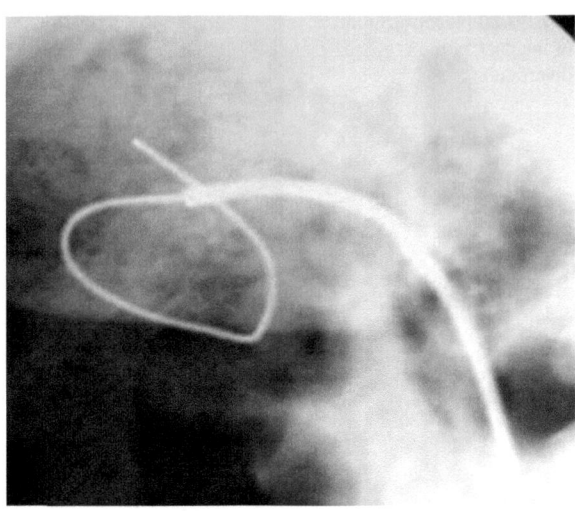

Fig. 20.23 Retrograde through scope

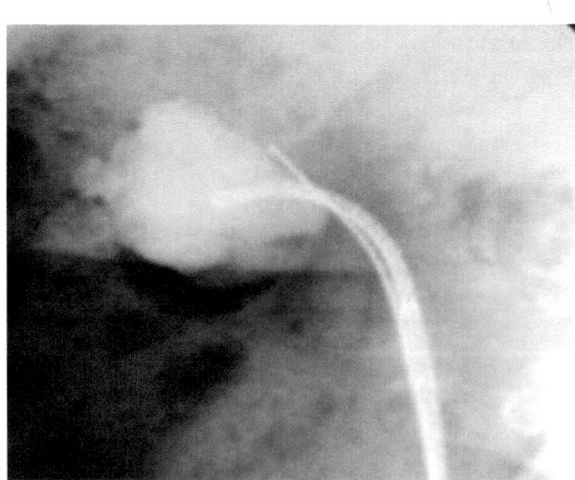

Fig. 20.24 Post
operative KUB

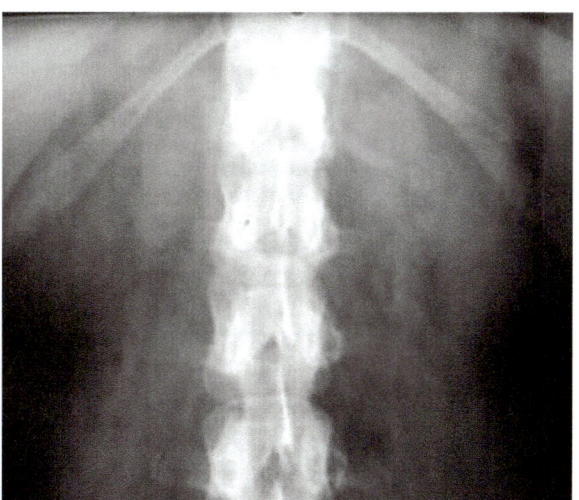

Minimally invasive procedure

Direct access to stone if upper /
mid calyx

Lower pole access difficult

Can incise / ablate neck of
diverticulum with holmium laser

Initial view into calyceal
diverticulum
Stone fragmentation
Incise infundibulum
Infundibulum open

The equipment

- Sensor wire 0.08 Fr- nitinol core over a hydrophilic coating
- Ureteric catheter- white (soft) or blue (stiffer)
- Contrast- Urograffin 150 or 300.
- Long rigid ureteroscope
- Flexible ureteroscope
- Access sheath

The strategy

- Rigid cystoscope in, with bridge
- Change to biopsy forceps
- Pass sensor to renal pelvis.
- Do a retrograde to see whether there are stones in the ureter
- Using the long rigid, do a diagnostic ureteroscopy. Alternatively if the ureter is clear on retrograde, railroad up a flexible ureteroscope.
- Identify the diverticulum, if necessary incise the neck and laser the stone
- Do not force the access sheath as the ureter can be tight
- 6x24 fr stent (female patient, shorter stent)

The difficulties

- Identifiying the diverticulum- sometimes it may be completely embedded in renal parenchyma
- When the diverticula neck is lasered, the can be bleeding, obstructing vision.
- If embedded fully in a calyceal diverticulum, it may not be cleared completely.
- Patients may often be asymptomatic - an operation may not be what these patients require

The outcome

- In this case, a flexible ureteroscopy was done identifying the calyceal neck.
- The infundibulum was incised and the stone lasered out
- 3months later the patient is asymptomatic

PNL should be considered as the primary modality for the management of symptomatic calyceal diverticula, especially in those patients with a large stone volume or lower pole location

URS may be considered in an initial attempt in patients with anteriorly located diverticula, or diverticula in the upper pole or mid portion of the kidney. Auge 2002.

20.10 Patient Information and Consent

Why is this procedure being done?

- This procedure is being done to remove stones from within an outpouching of the renal system
- It uses a camera through the bladder.
- The neck of the outpouching will be lasered open to get access to the stone
- This procedure is done with cameras to avoid more major operations such as open surgery for stone removal
- A stent will be required at the end of the procedure, which may be removed in a few days (stent on strings) or a couple of weeks using a camera (Flexible cystoscope)
- The procedure is done as a daycase and followup will be in at a routine outpatient appointment

What are the alternatives

- Conservative management
- ESWL-this is not an option as the stones will be unable to drain
- PCNL- using a camera through the back into the kidney, stones can be extracted
- Robotic or laparoscopic stone surgery- no commonly done for stones, but can be done for stones refractory to endoscopic management
- Open stone surgery- not commonly done for stones

What the procedure entails

- A general anaesthetic is used
- Antibiotics are given pre-procedure
- A camera is inserted and contrast studies are done
- A camera and laser will be passed to the kidney
- The stone will be broken to fragments or removed or dusted
- A stent will be passed up to the kidney that will be removed at a later date

The outcome

- Infection, sepsis, HDU/ ITU stay
- Bleeding
- Recurrence
- Remnant stone requiring further treatment
- Failure to reach stone requiring stenting and a 2nd look procedure or nephrostomy
- Trauma to the ureter- abrasion, stricture, mucosal damage, ureteric reconstruction
- Anaesthetic risks - MI, CVA, PE, DVT, Chest infection

References

Auge BK, Preminger GM. Update on shock wave lithotripsy technology. Curr Opin Urol. 2002;12(4):287–90.

Fuchs GJ, David RD, Fuchs AM. Complications of extracorporeal shockwave lithotripsy. Arch Esp Urol. 1989;42(Suppl 1):83–9.

Middleton AW Jr, Pfister RC. Stone-containing pyelocaliceal diverticulum: embryogenic, anatomic, radiologic and clinical characteristics. J Urol. 1974;111(1):2–6.

Psihramis KE, Dretler SP. Extracorporeal shock wave lithotripsy of caliceal diverticula calculi. J Urol. 1987;138(4):707–11.

Smyth N, Somani B, Rai B, Aboumarzouk OM. Treatment options for calyceal diverticula. Curr Urol Rep. 2019;20(7):37.

Streem SB, Yost A. Treatment of caliceal diverticular calculi with extracorporeal shock wave lithotripsy: patient selection and extended followup. J Urol. 1992;148(3 Pt 2):1043.

Timmons JW Jr, Malek RS, Hattery RR, Deweerd JH. Caliceal diverticulum. J Urol. 1975;114(1):6–9.

Williams G, Blandy JP, Tresidder GC. Communicating cysts and diverticula of the renal pelvis. Br J Urol. 1969;41(2):163–70.

Difficult Access to the Ureter

21.1 Manipulation of the Hostile Ureter

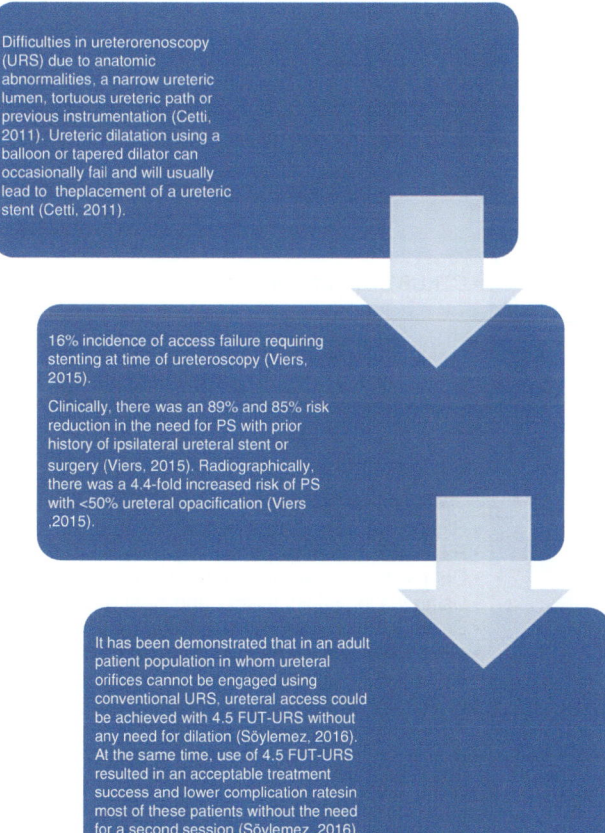

Difficulties in ureterorenoscopy (URS) due to anatomic abnormalities, a narrow ureteric lumen, tortuous ureteric path or previous instrumentation (Cetti, 2011). Ureteric dilatation using a balloon or tapered dilator can occasionally fail and will usually lead to theplacement of a ureteric stent (Cetti, 2011).

16% incidence of access failure requiring stenting at time of ureteroscopy (Viers, 2015).

Clinically, there was an 89% and 85% risk reduction in the need for PS with prior history of ipsilateral ureteral stent or surgery (Viers, 2015). Radiographically, there was a 4.4-fold increased risk of PS with <50% ureteral opacification (Viers ,2015).

It has been demonstrated that in an adult patient population in whom ureteral orifices cannot be engaged using conventional URS, ureteral access could be achieved with 4.5 FUT-URS without any need for dilation (Söylemez, 2016). At the same time, use of 4.5 FUT-URS resulted in an acceptable treatment success and lower complication ratesin most of these patients without the need for a second session (Söylemez, 2016).

S. S. Goonewardene et al., *Surgical Strategies in Endourology for Stone Disease*, https://doi.org/10.1007/978-3-030-82143-2_21

21.2   Case 1

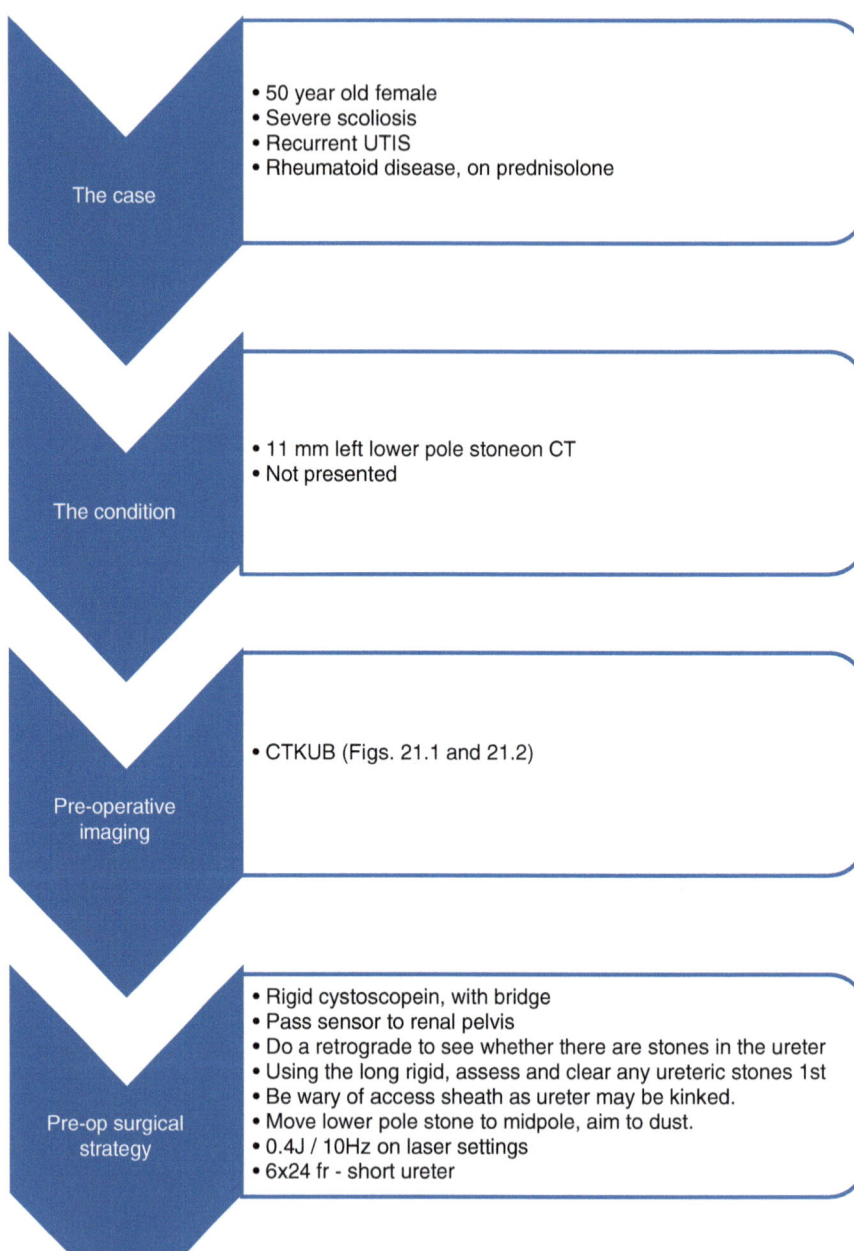

The case

- 50 year old female
- Severe scoliosis
- Recurrent UTIS
- Rheumatoid disease, on prednisolone

The condition

- 11 mm left lower pole stoneon CT
- Not presented

Pre-operative imaging

- CTKUB (Figs. 21.1 and 21.2)

Pre-op surgical strategy

- Rigid cystoscopein, with bridge
- Pass sensor to renal pelvis
- Do a retrograde to see whether there are stones in the ureter
- Using the long rigid, assess and clear any ureteric stones 1st
- Be wary of access sheath as ureter may be kinked.
- Move lower pole stone to midpole, aim to dust.
- 0.4J / 10Hz on laser settings
- 6x24 fr - short ureter

The equipment

- Sensor wire 0.08 Fr-nitinol core over a hydrophilic coating
- Ureteric catheter-white (soft) or blue (stiffer)
- Contrast- Urograffin 150 or 300.
- Long rigid ureteroscope
- FLexible ureteroscope
- Access sheath
- Xray and Laser

The strategy

- Rigid cystoscope in, with bridge
- Pass sensor to renal pelvis.
- Do a retrograde to see whether there are stones in the ureter
- Using the long rigid, do a diagnostic ureteroscopy to view all areas of the ureter
- Gauge the access sheath size very carefully, both length and diameter-35 long, 9/11/ fr wide
- If ureter clear identify renal pelvic stone. If in good position you may be able to laser with long rigid alone, but always have access sheath and flexible ureteroscopy on standby.
- Do not force the access sheath as the ureter can be tight
- 6x24 fr stent (female patient, shorter stent)

The difficulties

- Getting up past the kinks in a ureter-sometimes the sensor won't pass
- If this happens, use the blue ureteric catheter, which will stiffen the guidewire, or a terumo wire (very hydrophillic)
- Once the wire is past the kink, get a lot of wire into the renal pelvis-the automatic reflex of wire is to straighten and straighten out the kink.
- When passing up the long rigid ureteroscope, have a second wire as a probiscus to guide you.
- Poor vision-go for dusting over fragmentation.
- Use the washout technique to get rid of fragments

The outcome

- This patient was completely cleared of stone.

Fig. 21.1 Left lower pole renal stone 11 mm

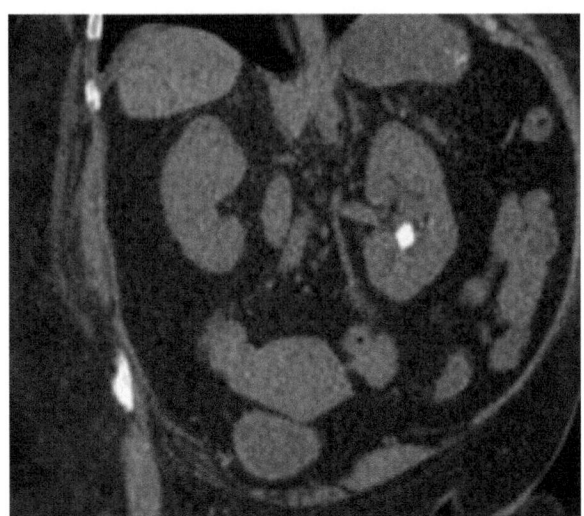

Fig. 21.2 Left lower pole renal stone

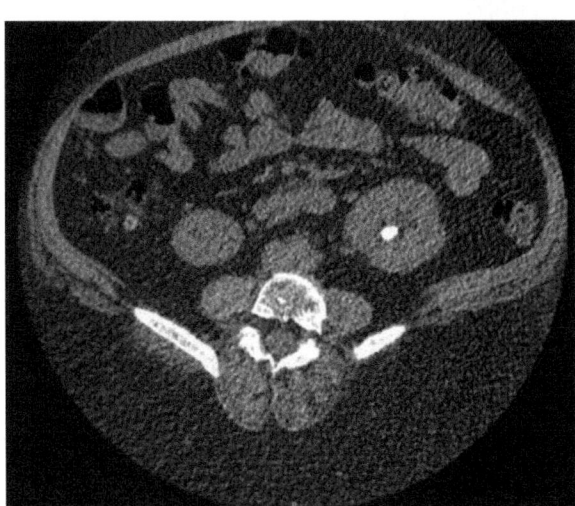

21.3 Patient Information and Consent: What to Tell the Patient

Why is this procedure being done?

- This procedure is being done to remove stones from the lower pole of the kidney using a camera through the bladder
- Stones are broken up using a laser
- This procedure is done with cameras to avoid more major operations such as open surgery for stone removal
- A stent will be required at the end of the procedure, which may be removed in a few days (stent on strings) or a couple of weeks using a camera (Flexible cystoscope)

What are the alternatives

- Conservative management
- ESWL-shock wave therapy to the stone to try and break it up-may require 2 sessions, f this fails, usually surgery is required
- PCNL-using a camera through the back into the kidney, very large stones can be extracted
- Robotic or laparoscopic stone surgery-no commonly done for stones
- Open stone surgery-not commonly done for stones

What the procedure entails

- A general anaesthetic is used
- Antibiotics are given pre-procedure
- A camera is inserted and constrast studies are done
- A camera and laser will be passed to the kidney
- The stone will be broken to fragments or removed or dusted
- A stent will be passed up to the kidney that will be removed at a later date

The outcome

- Infection, sepsis, HDU/ ITU stay
- Bleeding
- Recurrence
- Remnant stone requiring further treatment
- Failure to reach stone requiring stenting and a 2nd look procedure or nephrostomy
- Trauma to the ureter-abrasion, stricture, mucosal damage, ureteric reconstruction
- Anaesthetic risks-MI, CVA, PE, DVT, Chest infection

References

Cetti RJ, Biers S, Keoghane SR. The difficult ureter: what is the incidence of pre-stenting? Ann R Coll Surg Engl. 2011;93(1):31–3.

Söylemez H, Yıldırım K, Utangac MM, Aydoğan TB, Ezer M, Atar M. A new alternative for difficult ureter in adult patients: no need to dilate ureter via a balloon or a stent with the aid of 4.5F semirigid ureteroscope. J Endourol. 2016;30(6):650–4.

Viers BR, Viers LD, Hull NC, Hanson TJ, Mehta RA, Bergstralh EJ, Krambeck A, et al. The difficult ureter: clinical and radiographic characteristics associated with upper urinary tract access at the time of ureteroscopic stone treatment. Urology. 2015;86(5):878–84.

Surgical Strategy for an Encrusted Stent

22.1 Role of Biofilm Formation and Stent Encrustation

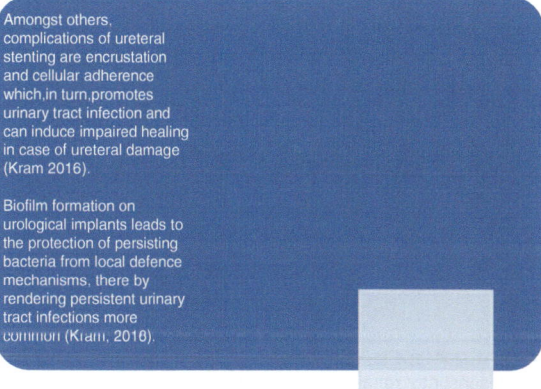

Amongst others, complications of ureteral stenting are encrustation and cellular adherence which, in turn, promotes urinary tract infection and can induce impaired healing in case of ureteral damage (Kram 2016).

Biofilm formation on urological implants leads to the protection of persisting bacteria from local defence mechanisms, there by rendering persistent urinary tract infections more common (Kram, 2016).

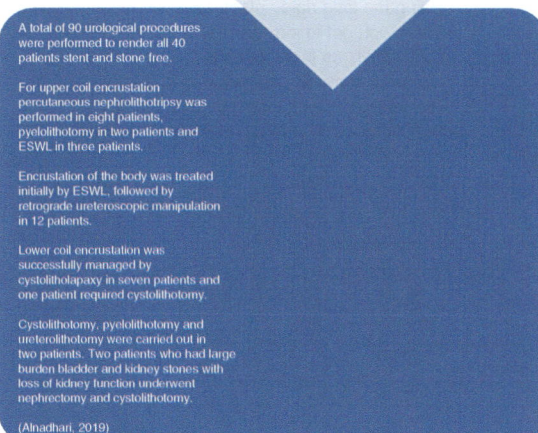

A total of 90 urological procedures were performed to render all 40 patients stent and stone free.

For upper coil encrustation percutaneous nephrolithotripsy was performed in eight patients, pyelolithotomy in two patients and ESWL in three patients.

Encrustation of the body was treated initially by ESWL, followed by retrograde ureteroscopic manipulation in 12 patients.

Lower coil encrustation was successfully managed by cystolitholapaxy in seven patients and one patient required cystolithotomy.

Cystolithotomy, pyelolithotomy and ureterolithotomy were carried out in two patients. Two patients who had large burden bladder and kidney stones with loss of kidney function underwent nephrectomy and cystolithotomy.

(Alnadhari, 2019)

S. S. Goonewardene et al., *Surgical Strategies in Endourology for Stone Disease*, https://doi.org/10.1007/978-3-030-82143-2_22

22.2   Case 1

The case
- 75year old male
- Stent in situ for 12 months
- Stroke patient
- Unable to communicate symptoms
- Non English speaker

The condition
- Encrusts incredibly quickly
- Stent left in situ for 4 weeks and had already started forming stone on both proximal and distal ureteric ends of stent
- Uric acid stone former previously

Pre-operative imaging
- CT KUB, XR KUB (Figs. 22.1, 22.2, 22.3 and 22.4)

Pre-op surgical strategy
- Rigid cystoscope in, with bridge
- Pass sensor to renal pelvis, coil and clip.
- If stone on end of stent, break off with biopsy forceps`
- Try to extract stent. If resistance, do not pull.
- Using the long rigid, place alongside stent and laser stone off as you find it.
- When you get to kidney, place 2nd wire and railroad flexible ureteroscope up
- 0.4J / 10Hz on laser settings
- Laser off stone at proximal end of stent
- Remove stent with stent removal forceps
- 6x26 fr on strings, remove at day 3 post op

Fig. 22.1 CT KUB stent
with encrustation

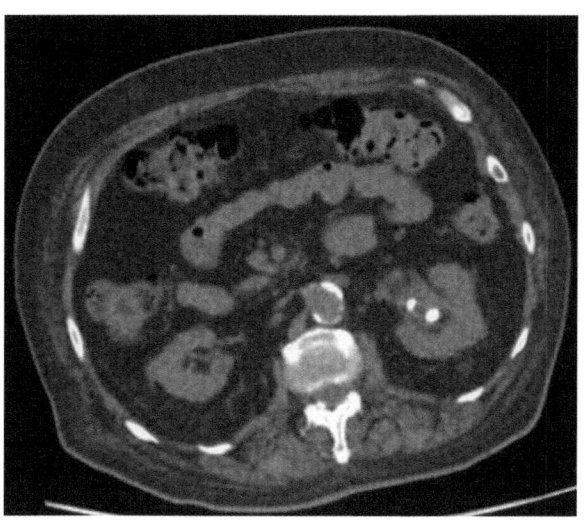

Fig. 22.2 Xray KUB
demonstrating stent

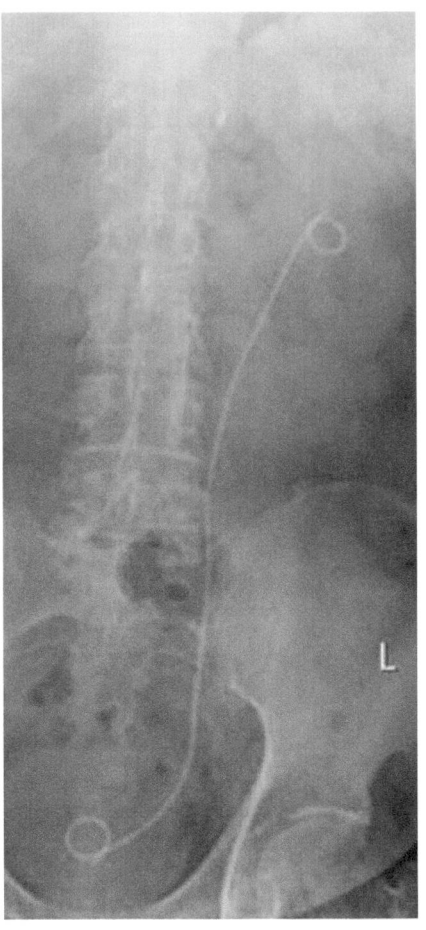

Fig. 22.3 Pyelogram from stent insertion

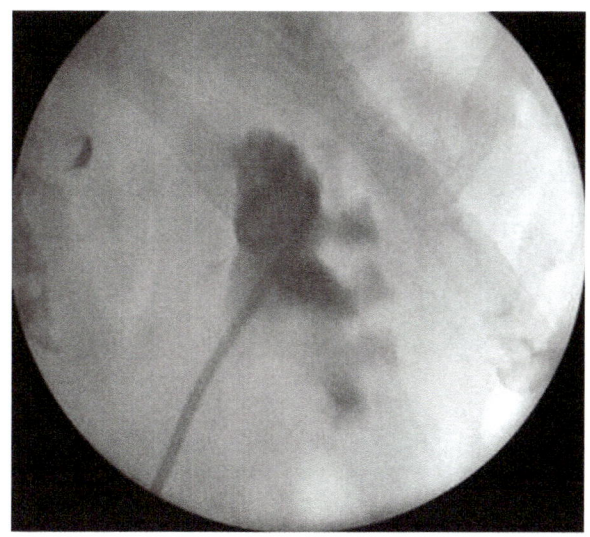

Fig. 22.4 Surgical strategy for an encrusted stent

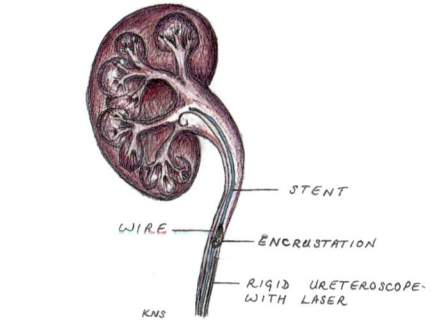

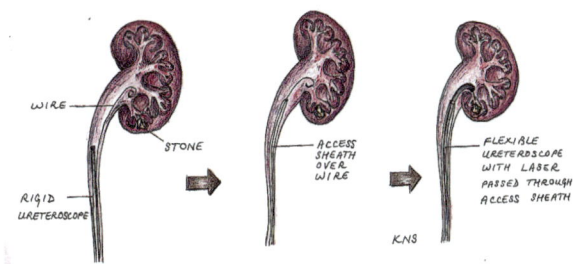

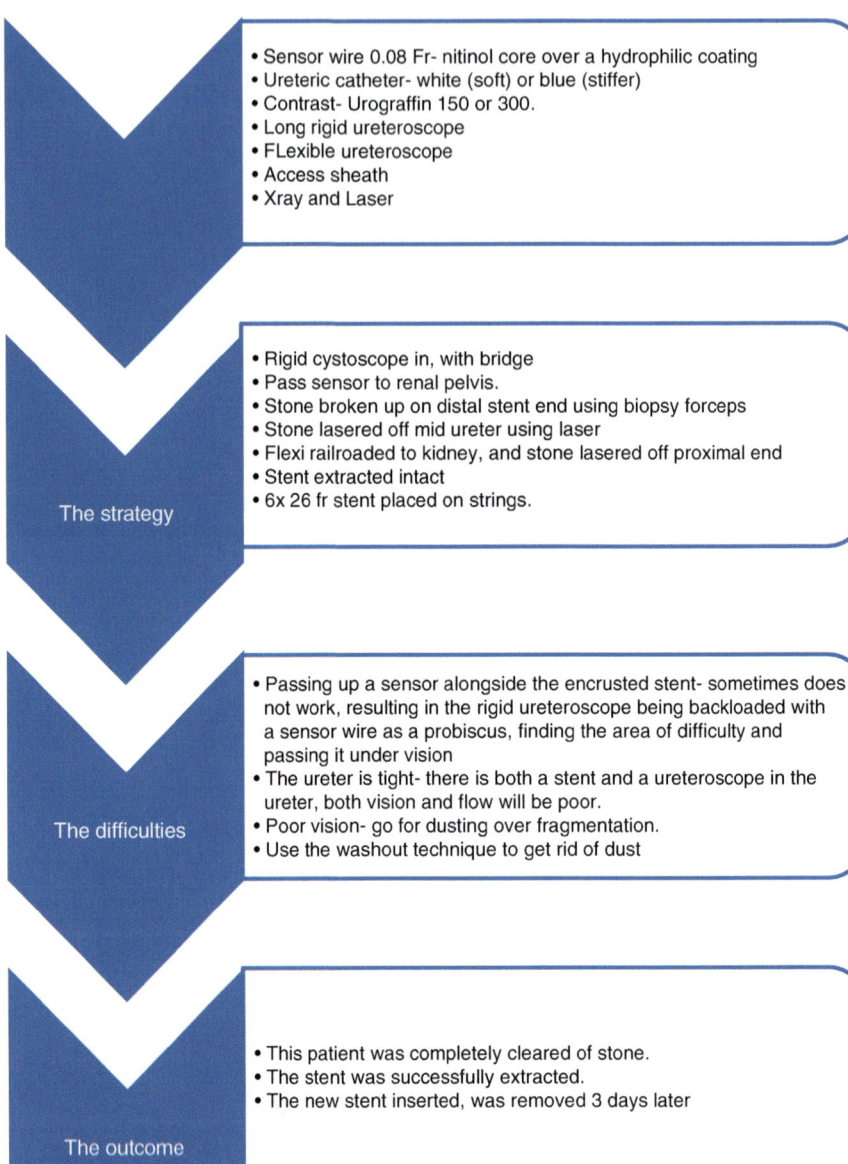

- Sensor wire 0.08 Fr- nitinol core over a hydrophilic coating
- Ureteric catheter- white (soft) or blue (stiffer)
- Contrast- Urograffin 150 or 300.
- Long rigid ureteroscope
- FLexible ureteroscope
- Access sheath
- Xray and Laser

The strategy

- Rigid cystoscope in, with bridge
- Pass sensor to renal pelvis.
- Stone broken up on distal stent end using biopsy forceps
- Stone lasered off mid ureter using laser
- Flexi railroaded to kidney, and stone lasered off proximal end
- Stent extracted intact
- 6x 26 fr stent placed on strings.

The difficulties

- Passing up a sensor alongside the encrusted stent- sometimes does not work, resulting in the rigid ureteroscope being backloaded with a sensor wire as a probiscus, finding the area of difficulty and passing it under vision
- The ureter is tight- there is both a stent and a ureteroscope in the ureter, both vision and flow will be poor.
- Poor vision- go for dusting over fragmentation.
- Use the washout technique to get rid of dust

The outcome

- This patient was completely cleared of stone.
- The stent was successfully extracted.
- The new stent inserted, was removed 3 days later

22.3 Patient Information and Consent: What to Tell the Patient

Why is this procedure being done?
- This procedure is being done to remove a stent with encrustation using a camera through the bladder
- Stones are broken up using a laser
- This procedure is done with cameras to avoid more major operations such as open surgery for stone removal
- A stent will be required at the end of the procedure, which may be removed in a few days (stent on strings).
- The follow up for this procedure will be a routine OPA

What are the alternatives
- ESWL- shock wave therapy, to the stone initially to try to break it up prior to surgery
- PCNL- using a camera through the back into the kidney, as part of an upper and lower approach to extracting the stent
- Robotic or laparoscopic stone surgery- not commonly done for encrusted stents
- Open stone surgery- not common done for encrusted stents

What the procedure entails
- A general anaesthetic is used
- Antibiotics are given pre-procedure
- A camera is inserted and contrast studies are done
- A camera and laser will be passed alongside the stent to remove encrustations using a laser
- The stone will be broken to fragments or removed or dusted
- A stent will be passed up to the kidney that will be removed in a few days

Side effects
- Infection, sepsis, HDU/ ITU stay
- Bleeding
- Recurrence
- Remnant stone/stent requiring further treatment
- Failure to reach stone/stent requiring stenting and a 2nd look procedure or nephrostomy
- Trauma to the ureter - abrasion, stricture, mucosal damage, ureteric reconstruction
- Anaesthetic risks - MI, CVA, PE, DVT, Chest infection

References

Alnadhari I, Alwan MA, Salah MA, Ghilan AM. Treatment of retained encrusted ureteral Double-J stent. Arch Ital Urol Androl. 2019;90(4):265–6.

Kram W, Buchholz N, Hakenberg OW. Ureteral stent encrustation. Pathophysiol Arch Esp Urol. 2016;69(8):485–93.

Surgical Strategy for Change of Ureteric Stents

23

23.1 Biofilm Formation in Stent Exchange

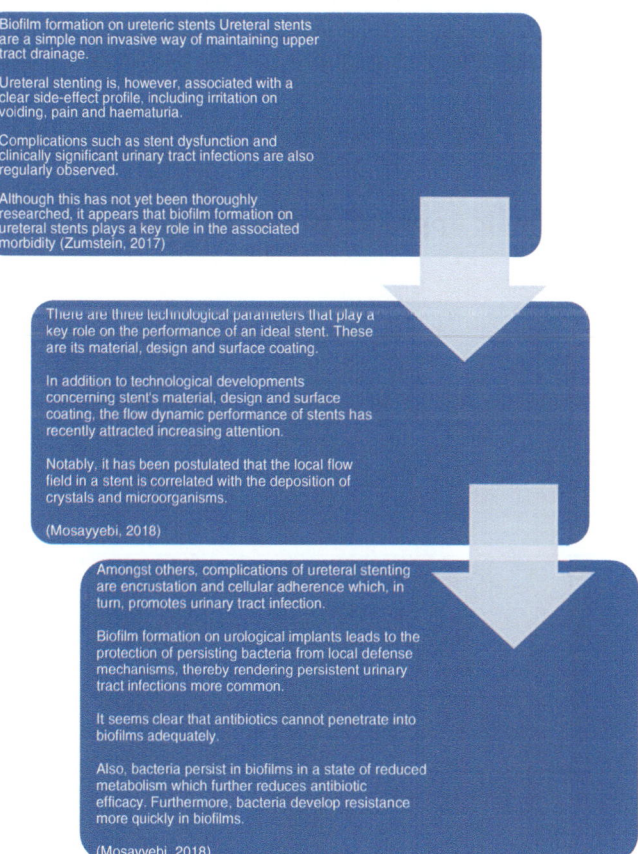

Biofilm formation on ureteric stents Ureteral stents are a simple non invasive way of maintaining upper tract drainage.

Ureteral stenting is, however, associated with a clear side-effect profile, including irritation on voiding, pain and haematuria.

Complications such as stent dysfunction and clinically significant urinary tract infections are also regularly observed.

Although this has not yet been thoroughly researched, it appears that biofilm formation on ureteral stents plays a key role in the associated morbidity (Zumstein, 2017)

There are three technological parameters that play a key role on the performance of an ideal stent. These are its material, design and surface coating.

In addition to technological developments concerning stent's material, design and surface coating, the flow dynamic performance of stents has recently attracted increasing attention.

Notably, it has been postulated that the local flow field in a stent is correlated with the deposition of crystals and microorganisms.

(Mosayyebi, 2018)

Amongst others, complications of ureteral stenting are encrustation and cellular adherence which, in turn, promotes urinary tract infection.

Biofilm formation on urological implants leads to the protection of persisting bacteria from local defense mechanisms, thereby rendering persistent urinary tract infections more common.

It seems clear that antibiotics cannot penetrate into biofilms adequately.

Also, bacteria persist in biofilms in a state of reduced metabolism which further reduces antibiotic efficacy. Furthermore, bacteria develop resistance more quickly in biofilms.

(Mosayyebi, 2018)

23.2   Case 1

The case
- 82 year old male
- Adenocarcinoma of prostate Gleason 3 + 3 in 12 / 12 cores, 90% maximum core involvement
- Presenting PSA 41,
- Bone scan negative
- Complete Brachy /radiotherapy, recent PSA 0.4

The condition
- Right sided hydronephrosis and dilated ureter down to bladder
- T3b N1 M0 prostate cancer

Pre-operative imaging
- CT Urogram
- Prior pyelogram
- Figures 23.1, 23.2, 23.3, 23.4, 23.5 and 23.6 for stenting equipment

The equipment

- Sensor wire 0.08 Fr- nitinol core over a hydrophilic coating
- Ureteric catheter- white (soft) or blue (stiffer)
- Contrast- Urograffin 150 or 300.
- Long rigid ureteroscope on standby
- Have Terumo wire and zebra wire on standby

The strategy

- Rigid cystoscope in, with bridge
- Pass sensor wire to renal pelvis.
- Screen stent out.
- Over guidewire railroad ureteric catheter
- Do a retrograde to assess position of renal pelvis
- Railroad 6x24 fr stent over guidewire

The difficulties

- If sensor wire fails to pass, pull stent to meatus with biopsy forceps and pass sensor through it to kidney.
- If that fails, pull stent out with biopsy forceps and try passing sensor up.
- If that does not work, try terumo (Very hydrophilic wire) or Reo wire.
- If that fails, get the long rigid ureteroscope , access ureter with sensor as a proboscis, visualise obstruction then pass wire under vision.
- Urethra- tight stricture in pre prostatic region- dilated with scope.
- Fixed pelvic floor due to prostate cancer.

The outcome

- Stent successfully inserted
- Stent register -completed.
- TCI card done for change of stent in 6 months.

Fig. 23.1 Right sided
hydronephrosis on CT
Urogram

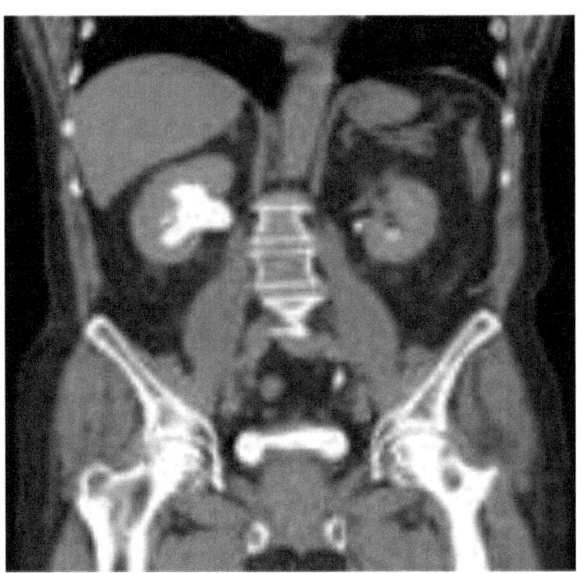

Fig. 23.2 Right sided
hydronephrosis on
pyelogram with sensor
wire up

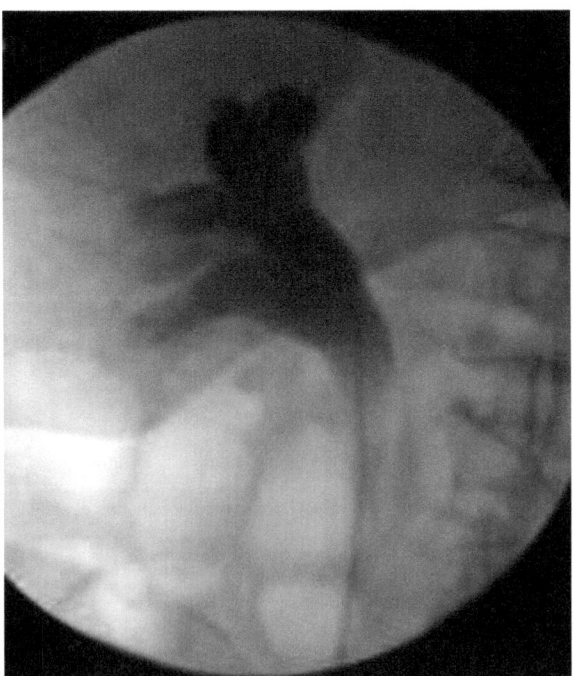

23.3   Outcomes with Stenting in Malignant Compression

Extrinsic malignant compression of the ureter is not uncommon, often refractory to decompression with conventional polymeric ureteral stents, and frequently associated with limited survival. (Elsamra, 2015). Alternative options for decompression include tandem ureteral stents, metallic stents and metal-mesh stents, though the preferred method remains controversial (Elsamra, 2015).

Elsamra reviewed outcomes with tandem ureteral stents for malignant ureteral obstruction, and carried out a PubMed search using the terms "malignant ureteral obstruction," "tandem ureteral stents," "ipsilateral ureteral stents," "metal ureteral stent," "resonance stent," "silhouette stent" and "metal mesh stent." (Elsamra, 2015).

Urinary tract infections have been associated with all stent types (Elsamra, 2015). A wide range of failure rates has been published for all types of stents, limiting direct comparison (Elsamra, 2015). Metal and metal-mesh stents show a high incidence of stent colic, migration and encrustation, whereas tandem stents appear to produce symptoms equivalent to single stents (Elsamra, 2015).

Comparison is difficult given the limited evidence and heterogeneity of patients with malignant ureteral obstruction. (Elsamra, 2015).

23.4   Patient Information and Consent: What to Tell Patients

Why is this procedure being done?

- This procedure is being done to change ureteric stents using a camera through the bladder
- Stones are broken up using a laser
- This procedure is done with cameras through the bladder
- A new stent will be inserted which will be changed in 6 months
- The follow up for this procedure will be a routine OPA
  What are

What are the alternatives

- Having a nephrostomy tube into the back
- Having an antegrade stent passed down a nephrostomy tube
- Having an extra - ureteric stent
- Having a memokath stent

What the procedure entails

- A general anaesthetic is used
- Antibiotics are given pre-procedure
- A camera is inserted and a wire passed up to the kidney
- The old stent will be removed
- A contrast study will be done
- A stent will be passed up to the kidney and changed in 6 months

Side effects

- Infection, sepsis, HDU/ ITU stay
- Bleeding
- Change of stent
- Stent related symptoms
- Failure, nephrostomy and antegrade stenting
- Trauma to the ureter- abrasion, stricture, mucosal damage, ureteric reconstruction
- Anaesthetic risks - MI, CVA, PE, DVT, Chest infection

The Albarran bridge allows downward and upward deflection of a guidewire prior to stent placement.

Fig. 23.3 A ureteric stent (the Double J Stent)

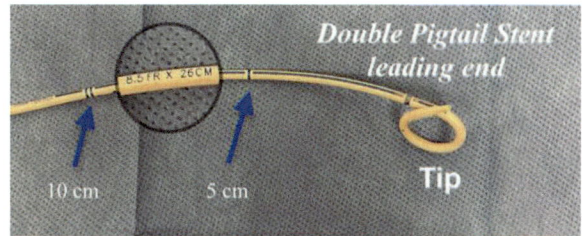

Fig. 23.4 A ureteric catheter for retrograde studies

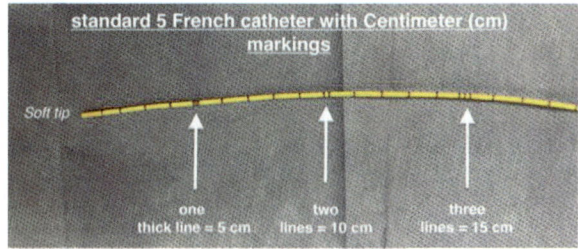

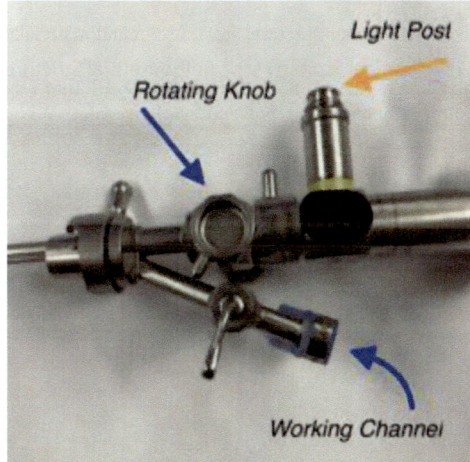

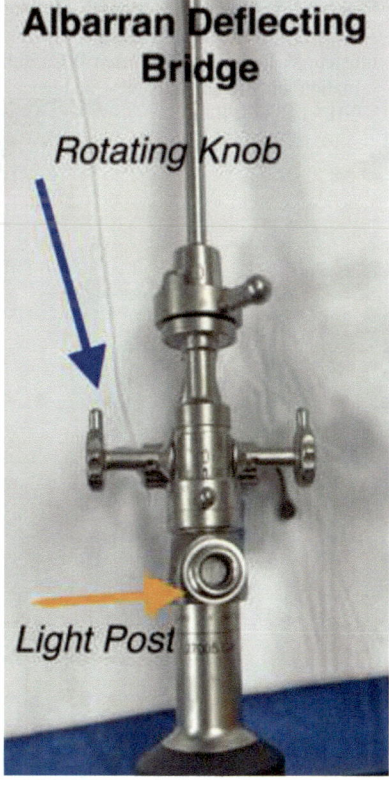

Fig. 23.5 The Albarran deflecting bridge

Fig. 23.6 Deflection of the Albarran Bridge

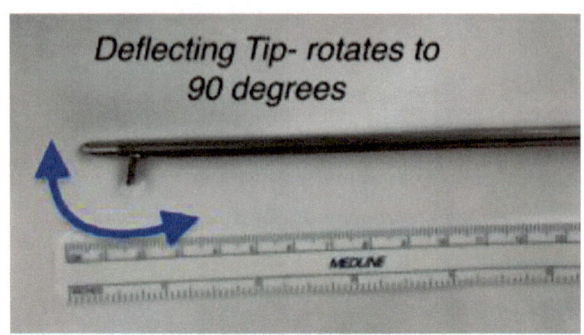

References

Elsamra SE, Leavitt DA, Motato HA, Friedlander JI, Siev M, Keheila M, Hoenig DM, Smith AD, Okeke Z. Stenting for malignant ureteral obstruction: tandem, metal or metal-mesh stents. Int J Urol. 2015;22(7):629–36.

Kram W, Buchholz N, Hakenberg OW. Ureteral stent encrustation. Pathophysiol Arch Esp Urol. 2016;69(8):485–93.

Mosayyebi A, Manes C, Carugo D, Somani BK. Advances in ureteral stent design and materials. Curr Urol Rep. 2018;19(5):35.

Zumstein V, Betschart P, Albrich WC, Buhmann MT, Ren Q, Schmid H-P, Abt D. Biofilm formation on ureteral stents – incidence, clinical impact, and prevention. Swiss Med Wkly. 2017;147:w14408.

Surgical Strategy for Bilateral Renal Stones

24.1 Bilateral Single Stone Endoscopic Procedures

Bilateral single stone endoscopic procedures

Bilateral single-session endoscopic procedures for bilateral renal stones are effective and safe.

Key to success is the proper selection of patients and extending surgery on the second side only when the first side has been uneventful. (Proietti, 2017)

Proetti conducted a SR into use of bilateral FURS.

Postoperative complications were mostly described as minor complications; one major complication (0.5%) (grade V) was reported.

The primary SFR ranged from 24% to 100%.

In all the studies a total of 29 (4%) major complications were described: 28 of them grade III while one was grade IV. One single study of bilateral PCNL with contralateral FURS for renal stones was identified.

24.2 Management of Bilateral Complex Renal Stones

The treatment of bilateral complex renal stones is a tough challenge for urologists (Liang, 2017). This study aimed to evaluate the efficiency and safety of bilateral ultrasonography-guided multi-tract percutaneous nephrolithotomy (PCNL) combined with EMS lithotripsy for the treatment of such cases (Liang, 2017). Twenty-seven patients suffering from bilateral complex renal calculi underwent t bilateral multi-tract PCNL (Liang, 2017).

The PCNL began with the establishment of percutaneous nephrostomy access, which was achieved under ultrasound guidance followed by stone fragment and removal by EMS lithotripsy (Liang, 2017). The same processes were then performed on the ipsilateral and contralateral renal units until the operation terminated (Liang, 2017). Sheaths left in situ to provide the tracts for the twostage and the three-stage PCNL procedures.

Renal stones of both sides were completely cleared within three PCNL sessions in 24 cases (Liang, 2017). Among them, four, thirteen, and seven cases underwent single, second-stage and third-stage procedures, respectively (Liang, 2017). The total stone-free rate was 88.9%. Three patients failed to receive complete stone clearance. Mean operation time was 78.7 (26-124) min, the mean estimated blood loss was 97.3 (30-250) ml, and the mean length of hospital stay was 18 (10-31) days (Liang, 2017). No patient required blood transfusion and postoperative fever occurred in 6 cases. Within the follow-up period, stone recurrence occurred in 6 patients (Liang, 2017).

Ultrasonography-guided multi-tract PCNL using EMS is an efficient method for the treatment of complex renal calculi (Liang, 2017). According to our experience, it is safe to make multiple tracts on both sides simultaneously (Liang, 2017).

24.3   Case 1

The case
- 40 year old female
- Presumed previous parathyroidectomy
- 2 prior URS, recurrent stone former prior to parathyroidectomy

The condition
- 6mm distal left ureteric stone
- Left ureteric stone and multiple bilateral renal stones with nephrocalcinosis
- Not presented

Pre-operative imaging
- CT KUB (Figs. 24.1 and 24.2)

Pre-op surgical strategy
- Clear the left side 1st and stent, prior to clearing the right side
- Rigid cystoscope in, with bridge
- Pass sensor to renal pelvis, coil and clip
- Do a retrograde to identify ureteric stone.
- Using the long rigid, identify, laser and extract stone-in ureter fragment and extract.
- Go up to renal pelvis and ensure ureter clear, retrograde via ureteroscope to map renal pelvis and stones.
- Calibrate ureter, and pass access sheath, 35 long 9/11 or 10/12
- 6x24 fr stent

The equipment

- Sensor wire 0.08 Fr- nitinol core over a hydrophilic coating
- Ureteric catheter- white (soft) or blue (stiffer)
- Contrast- Urograffin 150 or 300.
- Long rigid ureteroscope
- Flexible ureteroscope
- Access sheath - depending on urethral calibration- 45 long 9/12 or 45 long10/12.

The strategy

- Rigid cystoscope in, with bridge
- Recurrence noted in bladder-
- Pass sensor to renal pelvis.
- URS allowed clearance of left distal ureteric stone.
- Access sheath 35 long, 10/12 fr was passed to renal pelvis.
- 6x24 fr stent (female patient, shorter stent)

The difficulties

- Clearing the ureter properly first, to allow an access sheath to - passoften the ureter is thin and friable.
- Nephrocalcinosis may often mean there are no renal stones within the calyces
- If the stone burden is heavy, a 2nd operation may be required.
- Poor vision and debris- keep movements small and microscopic.

The outcome

- The patient had the left side cleared first, then was brought back for a 2nd right sided procedure
- Post operatively, the stent was tracked as part of a stent register
- BAUS dietary advice was given

Fig. 24.1 Patient with
bilateral renal stones

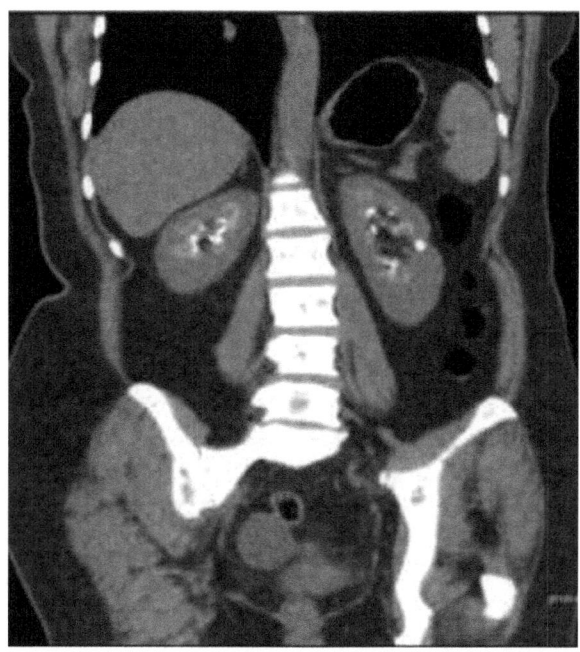

Fig. 24.2 Distal left
ureteric stone

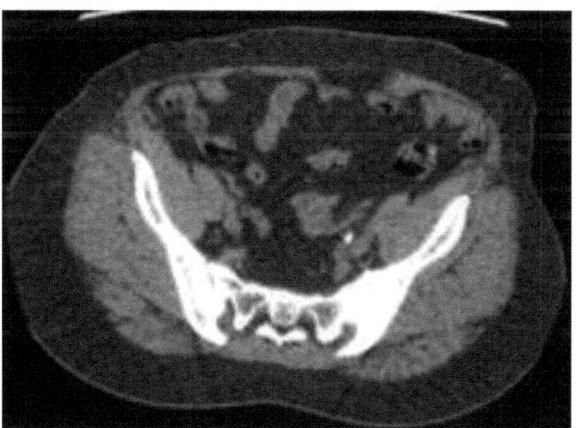

24.4   Patient Information and Consent: What to Tell the Patient

Why is this procedure being done?

- This procedure is being done to remove stones from within the kidney using a camera through the bladder
- As stones are present on both sides, one side will be cleared first, then the other.
- Stones are broken up using a laser
- This procedure is done with cameras to avoid more major operations such as open surgery for stone removal
- A stent will be required at the end of the procedure, which may be removed in a few days (stent on strings) or a couple of weeks using a camera (Flexible cystoscope)
- The procedure is done as a daycase and followup will be in at a routine outpatient appointment

What are the alternatives

- Conservative management - this is unlikely as stone can move and block each kidney
- ESWL- this tends to be unlikely as both sides need to be cleared
- PCNL- using a camera through the back into the kidney, very large stones can be extracted
- Robotic or laparoscopic stone surgery- no commonly done for stones
- Open stone surgery- not common done for stones

What the procedure entails

- A general anaesthetic is used
- Antibiotics are given pre-procedure
- A camera is inserted and contrast studies are done
- A camera and laser will be passed to the kidney
- The stone will be broken to fragments or removed or dusted
- A stent will be passed up to the kidney that will be removed at a later date.
- The other kidney may also be stented to protect drainage

The outcome

- Infection, sepsis, HDU/ ITU stay
- Bleeding
- Recurrence
- Remnant stone requiring further treatment
- Failure to reach stone requiring stenting and a 2nd look procedure or nephrostomy
- Trauma to the ureter- abrasion, stricture, mucosal damage, ureteric reconstruction
- Anaesthetic risks - MI, CVA, PE, DVT, Chest infection

References

Proietti S, de la Rosette J, Eisner B, Gaboardi F, Fiori C, Kinzikeeva E, Luciani L, Miano R, Porpiglia F, Rosso M, Sofer M, Traxer O, Giusti G. Minerva. Urol Nefrol. 2017;69(5):432–45.

Liang T, Zhao C, Wu G, Tang B, Luo X, Lu S, Yu D, Yang H. Multi-tract percutaneous nephrolithotomy combined with EMS lithotripsy for bilateral complex renal stones: our experience. BMC Urol. 2017;17(1):15.

Surgical Strategy for Ureteric Strictures

25

25.1 Preoperative Evaluation and Management Options

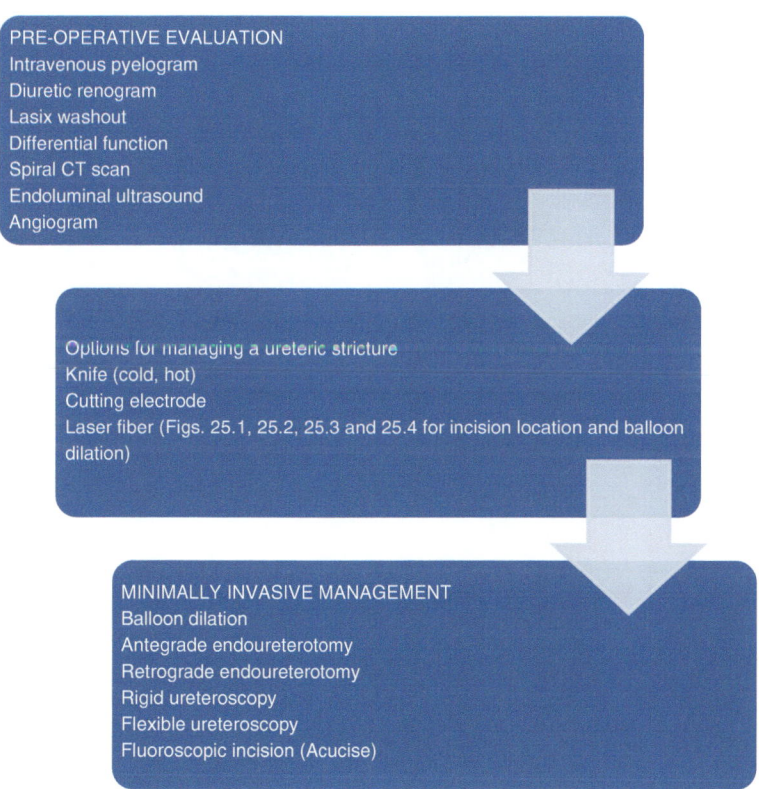

PRE-OPERATIVE EVALUATION
Intravenous pyelogram
Diuretic renogram
Lasix washout
Differential function
Spiral CT scan
Endoluminal ultrasound
Angiogram

Options for managing a ureteric stricture
Knife (cold, hot)
Cutting electrode
Laser fiber (Figs. 25.1, 25.2, 25.3 and 25.4 for incision location and balloon dilation)

MINIMALLY INVASIVE MANAGEMENT
Balloon dilation
Antegrade endoureterotomy
Retrograde endoureterotomy
Rigid ureteroscopy
Flexible ureteroscopy
Fluoroscopic incision (Acucise)

Fig. 25.1 Incision
location

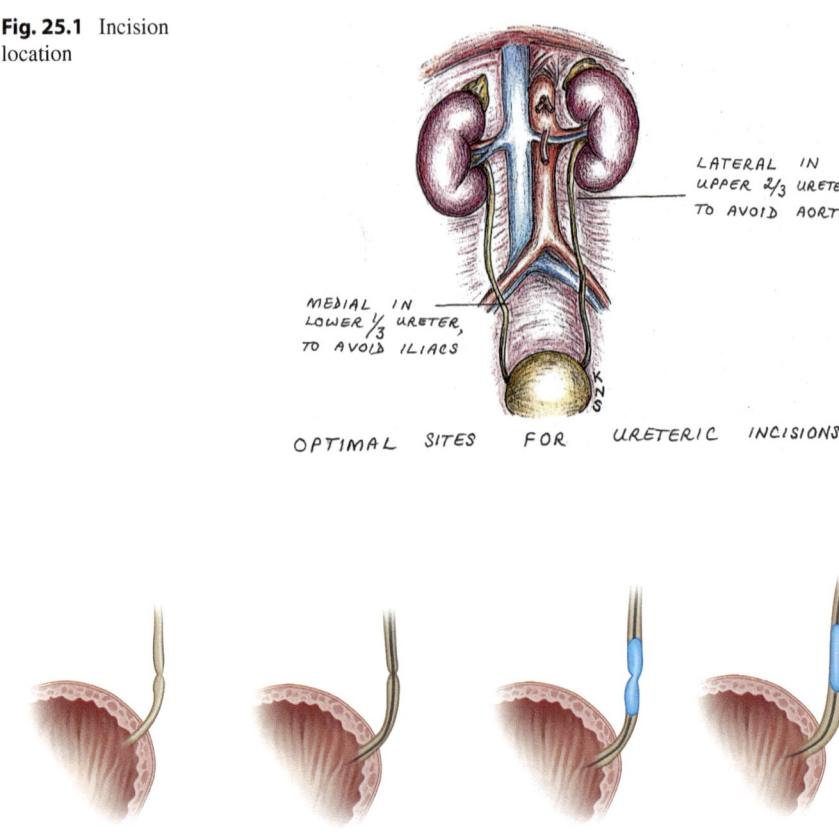

LATERAL   IN
UPPER 2/3 URETER,
TO AVOID AORTA

MEDIAL   IN
LOWER 1/3 URETER,
TO AVOID ILIACS

OPTIMAL   SITES   FOR   URETERIC   INCISIONS

Ballon dilatation of ureteric stricture over a guide wire

Fig. 25.2 Balloon dilation of a ureteric stricture over a guidewire

Fig. 25.3 Balloon dilation

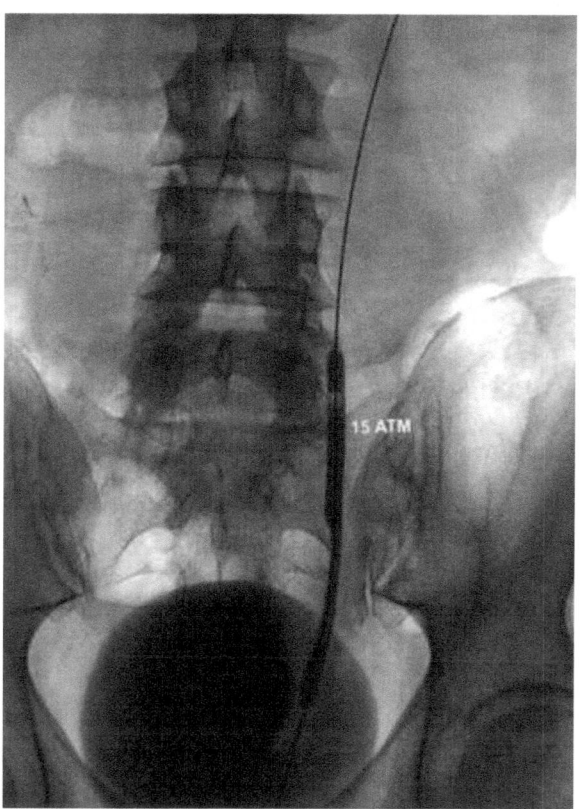

Fig. 25.4 Results of
balloon dilation—overall
success 50%

Study	Date	Size	Success
Banner	1983	12Fr	48%
Glanz	1983	12Fr	33%
Banner	1984	12Fr	48%
Finnerty	1984	12Fr	83%
Chang	1987	15 -24Fr	63%
O'Brien	1988	12-28Fr	50%

25.2 Case 1 Balloon Dilation of a Ureteric Stricture

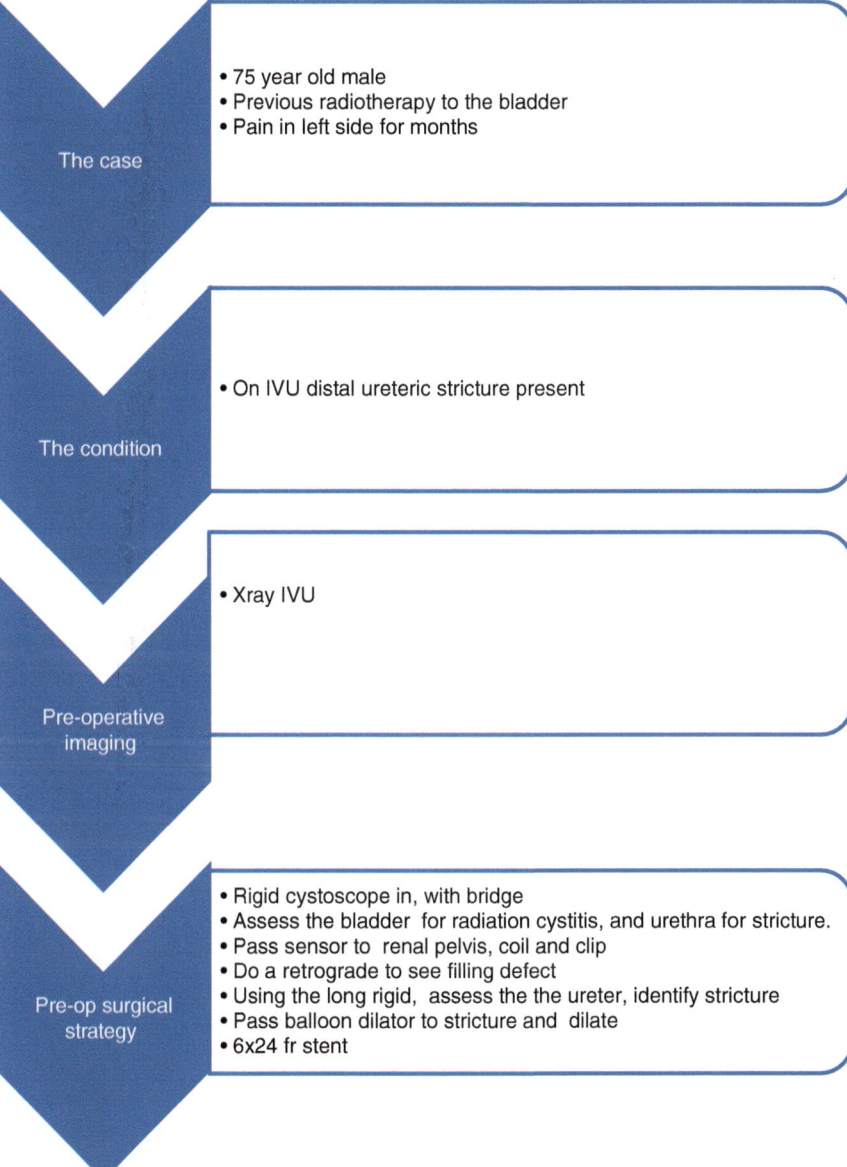

The case
- 75 year old male
- Previous radiotherapy to the bladder
- Pain in left side for months

The condition
- On IVU distal ureteric stricture present

Pre-operative imaging
- Xray IVU

Pre-op surgical strategy
- Rigid cystoscope in, with bridge
- Assess the bladder for radiation cystitis, and urethra for stricture.
- Pass sensor to renal pelvis, coil and clip
- Do a retrograde to see filling defect
- Using the long rigid, assess the the ureter, identify stricture
- Pass balloon dilator to stricture and dilate
- 6x24 fr stent

The equipment

- Sensor wire 0.08 Fr- nitinol core over a hydrophilic coating
- Balloon dilator
- Ureteric catheter- white (soft) or blue (stiffer)
- Contrast- Urograffin 150 or 300.
- Long rigid ureteroscope

The strategy

- Rigid cystoscope in, with bridge, pass sensor to renal pelvis.
- Pass rigid ureteroscope to stricture and do retrograde
- Assess length of stricture
- Pass balloon dilator into position and dilate stricture
- 6x26 fr stent (male patient, longer stent)

The difficulties

- Gettng the sensor wire past the stricture
- If that fails, railroad it through the ureteric catheter and use that as a platform
- Otherwise, use the rigid ureteroscope to identify the stricture and pass the guidewire under vision
- Getting the balloon dilator into place - be very gentle.
- Alternative options- use the holmium laser through the ureteroscope

The outcome

- After this patient had the stent removed, the MAG 3 renogram did not demonstrate any evidence of obstruction

25.3   Case 2 Holmium Laser Incision for a Distal Ureteric Stricture

The case

- 65 year old male
- Previous brachytherapy to the prostate
- Pain in left side and recurrent UTIs

The condition

- On IVU distal ureteric stricture present

Pre-operative imaging

- Xray IVU (Fig. 25.5)

Pre-op surgical strategy

- Rigid cystoscope in, with bridge (Figs. 25.6, 25.7, 25.8 and 25.9)
- Assess the bladder for radiation cystitis, and urethra for stricture
- Pass sensor to renal pelvis, coil and clip
- Do a retrograde to see filling defect
- Using the long rigid, assess the ureter, identify stricture
- Pass holmium laser up through scope and laser medially - stricture in distal third of ureter
- 6x24 fr stent

The equipment

- Sensor wire 0.08 Fr- nitinol core over a hydrophilic coating
- Balloon dilator
- Ureteric catheter- white (soft) or blue (stiffer)
- Contrast- Urograffin 150 or 300.
- Long rigid ureteroscope

The strategy

- Rigid cystoscope in, with bridge, pass sensor to renal pelvis
- Pass rigid ureteroscope to stricture and do retrograde
- Assess length of stricture
- Pass balloon dilator into position and dilate stricture
- 6x26 fr stent (male patient, longer stent)

The difficulties

- Gettng the sensor wire past the stricture
- If that fails, railroad it through the ureteric catheter and use that as a platform
- Otherwise, use the rigid ureteroscope to identify the stricture and pass the guidewire under vision
- When lasering starts, vision can go easily

The outcome

- After this patient had the stent removed, the IVP did not demonstrate any evidence of obstruction

Fig. 25.5 Retrograde
demonstrating stricture

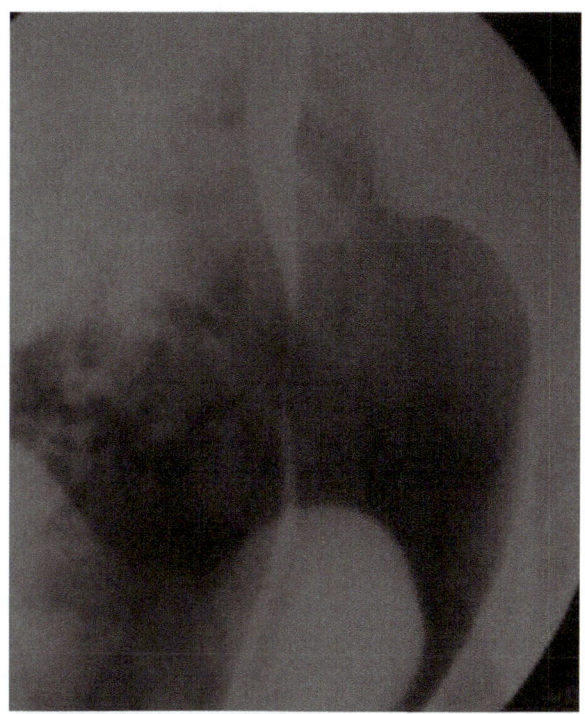

Fig. 25.6 Mark level of
stricture using fluoroscopy

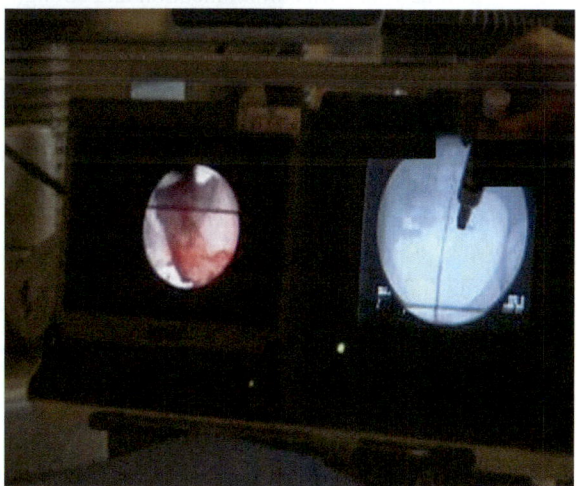

Fig. 25.7 Placement of
guidewire

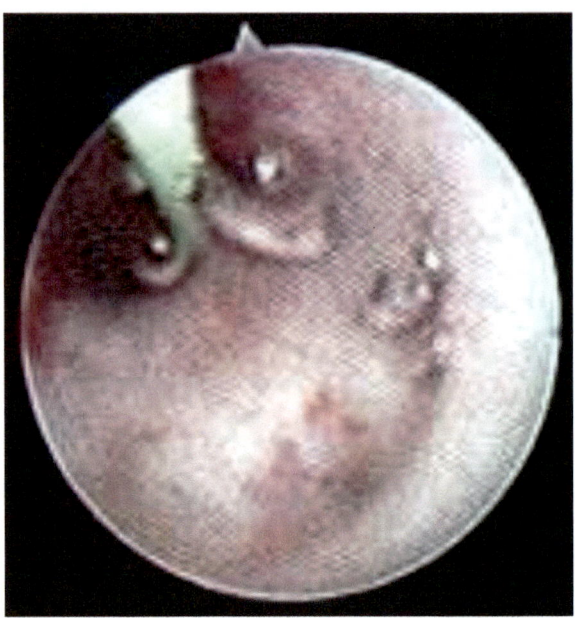

Fig. 25.8 Holmium laser
up to stricture

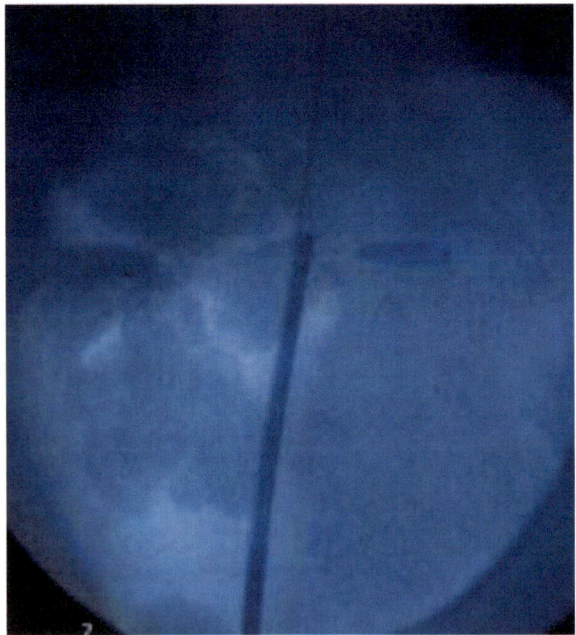

Fig. 25.9 Post op IVP

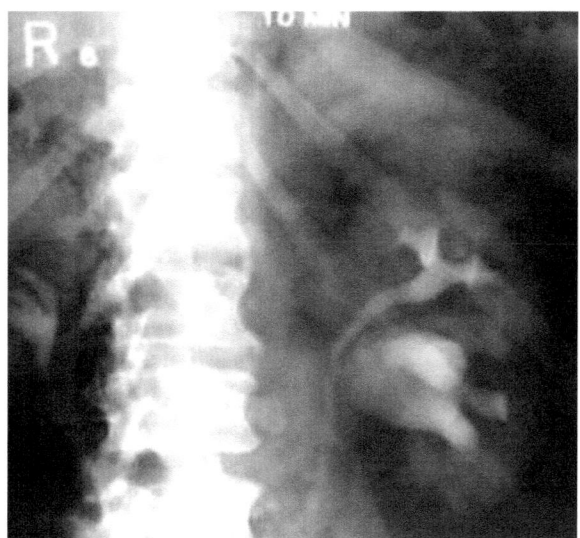

25.4   Case 3 Management of a Ureteric Stricture with a Cutting Balloon

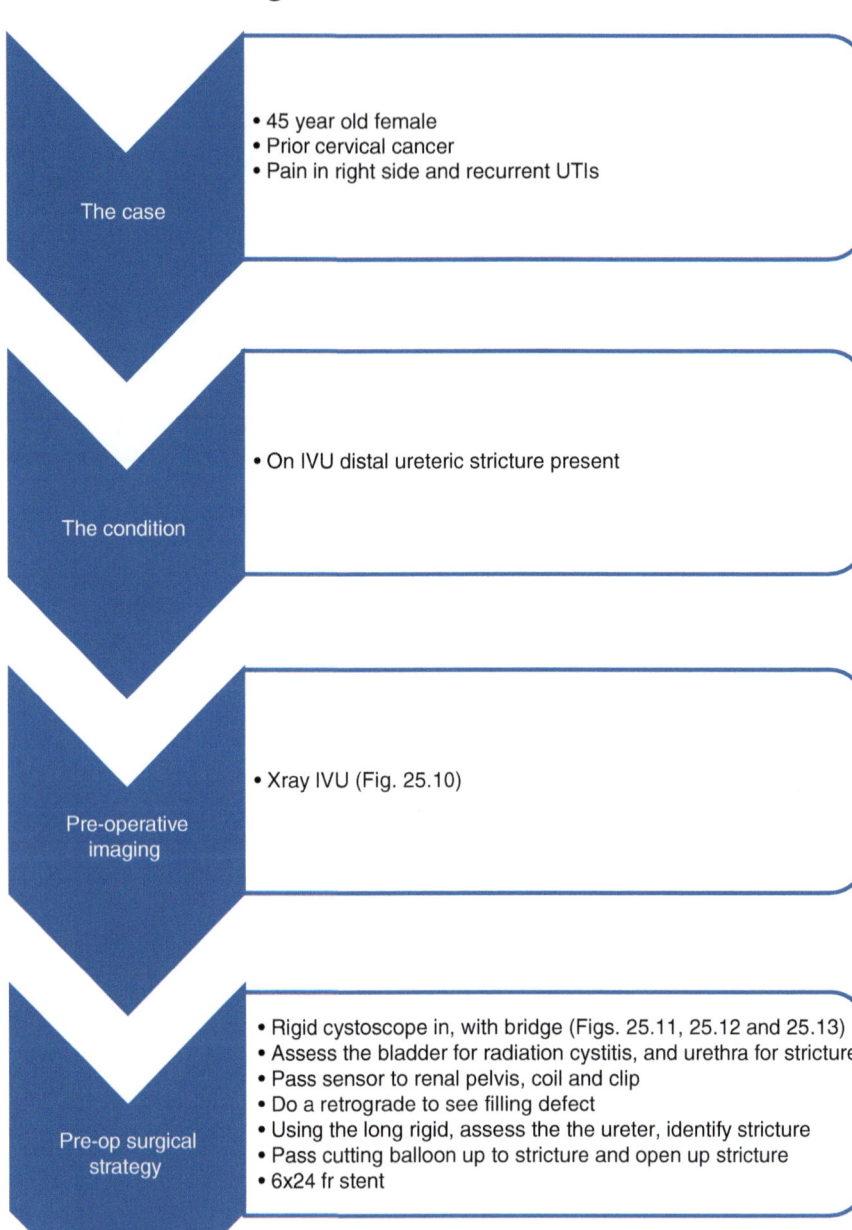

The case

- 45 year old female
- Prior cervical cancer
- Pain in right side and recurrent UTIs

The condition

- On IVU distal ureteric stricture present

Pre-operative imaging

- Xray IVU (Fig. 25.10)

Pre-op surgical strategy

- Rigid cystoscope in, with bridge (Figs. 25.11, 25.12 and 25.13)
- Assess the bladder for radiation cystitis, and urethra for stricture.
- Pass sensor to renal pelvis, coil and clip
- Do a retrograde to see filling defect
- Using the long rigid, assess the the ureter, identify stricture
- Pass cutting balloon up to stricture and open up stricture
- 6x24 fr stent

Benign Ureteral Strictures:
> Failures appear within 1 year
> Repeat endoureterotomy has high likelihood of success (if radiological improvement noted)

Ureteroenteric Strictures:
> Failures continue for first 3 years
> Repeat incisions likely to fail

Uniformly poor results when renal function < 25%

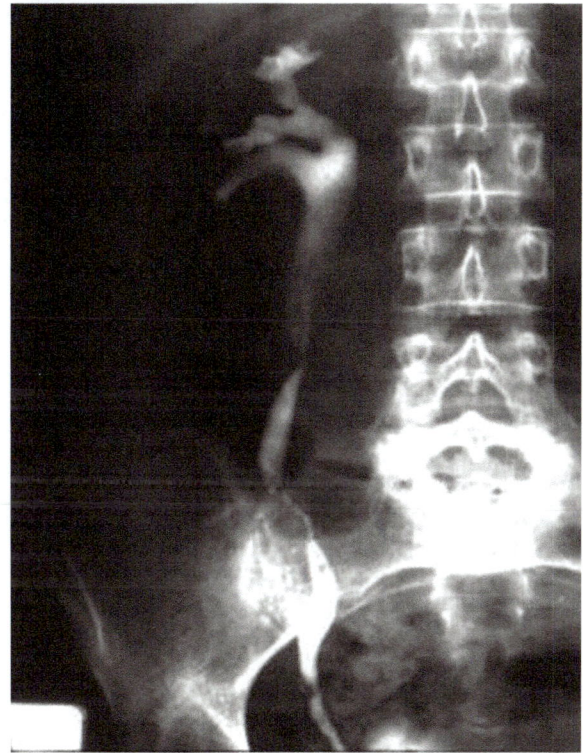

Fig. 25.10 Pre-operative IVU

Fig. 25.11 Balloon
placement across stricture

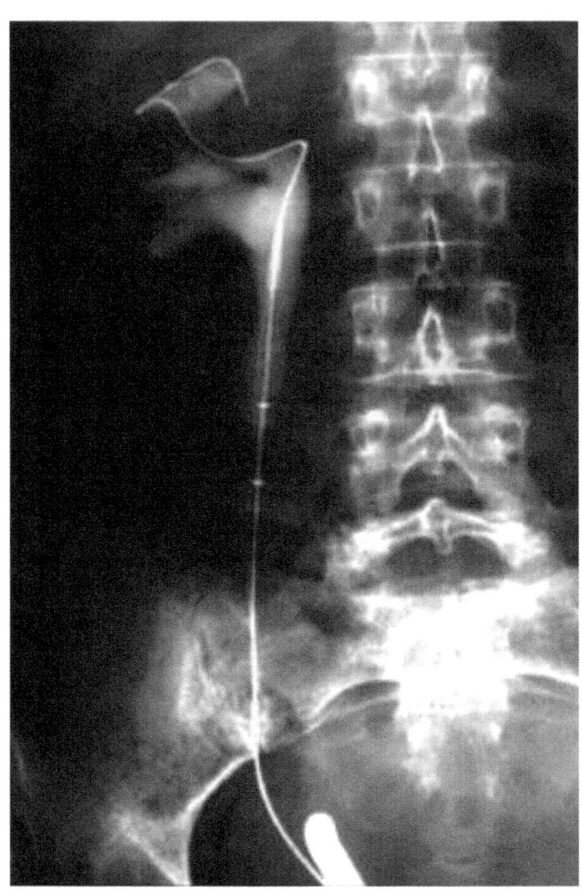

Fig. 25.12 Cutting
stricture and dilating
balloon

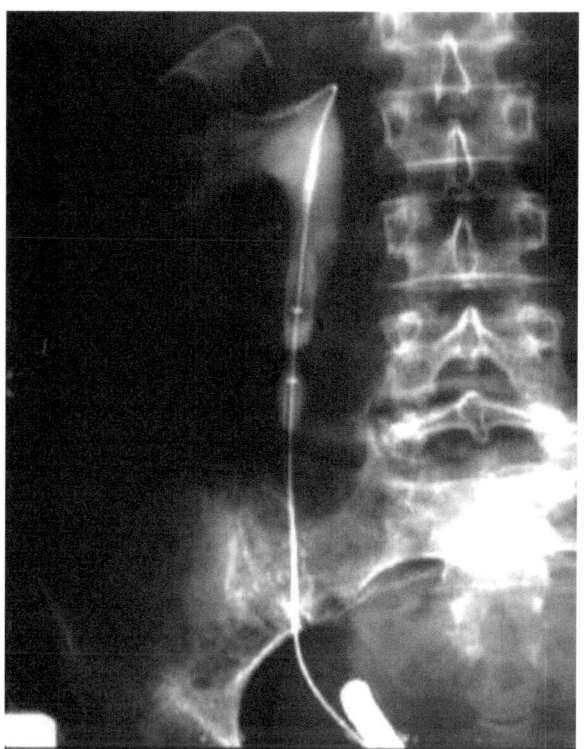

Fig. 25.13 Post op stent in position

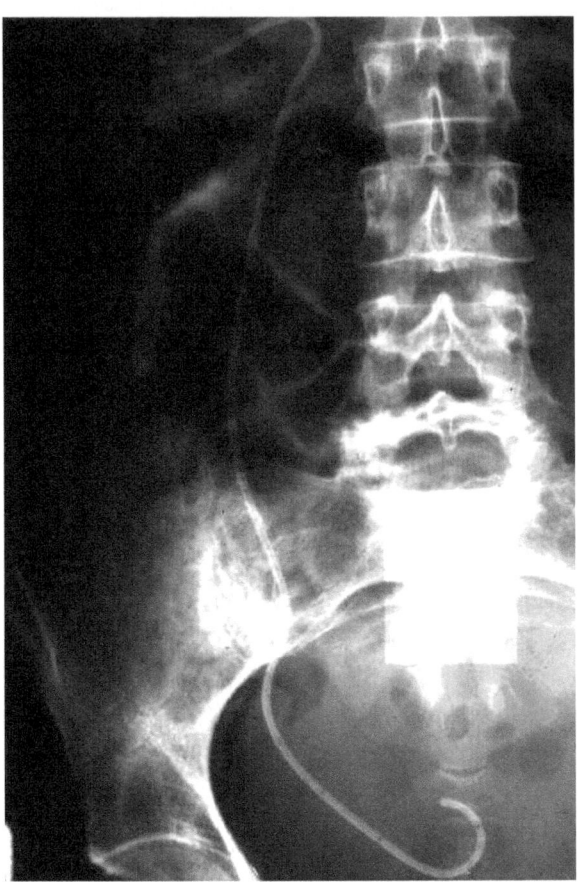

The equipment

- Sensor wire 0.08 Fr- nitinol core over a hydrophilic coating
- Cutting balloon
- Ureteric catheter- white (soft) or blue (stiffer)
- Contrast- Urograffin 150 or 300.
- Long rigid ureteroscope

The strategy

- Rigid cystoscope in, with bridge, pass sensor to renal pelvis.
- Pass rigid ureteroscope to stricture and do retrograde
- Assess length of stricture
- Pass balloon dilator into position and dilate stricture
- 6x24 fr stent (female patient, longer stent)

The difficulties

- Getting the sensor wire past the stricture
- If that fails, railroad it through the ureteric catheter and use that as a platform
- Otherwise, use the rigid ureteroscope to identify the stricture and passthe guidewire under vision
- As soon as you start cutting the stricture, bleeding may start and vision may go

The outcome

- After this patient had the stent removed, the IVP did not demonstrate any evidence of obstruction

25.5   Case 4 Management of a Ureteric Stricture with an Antegrade and Retrograde Approach

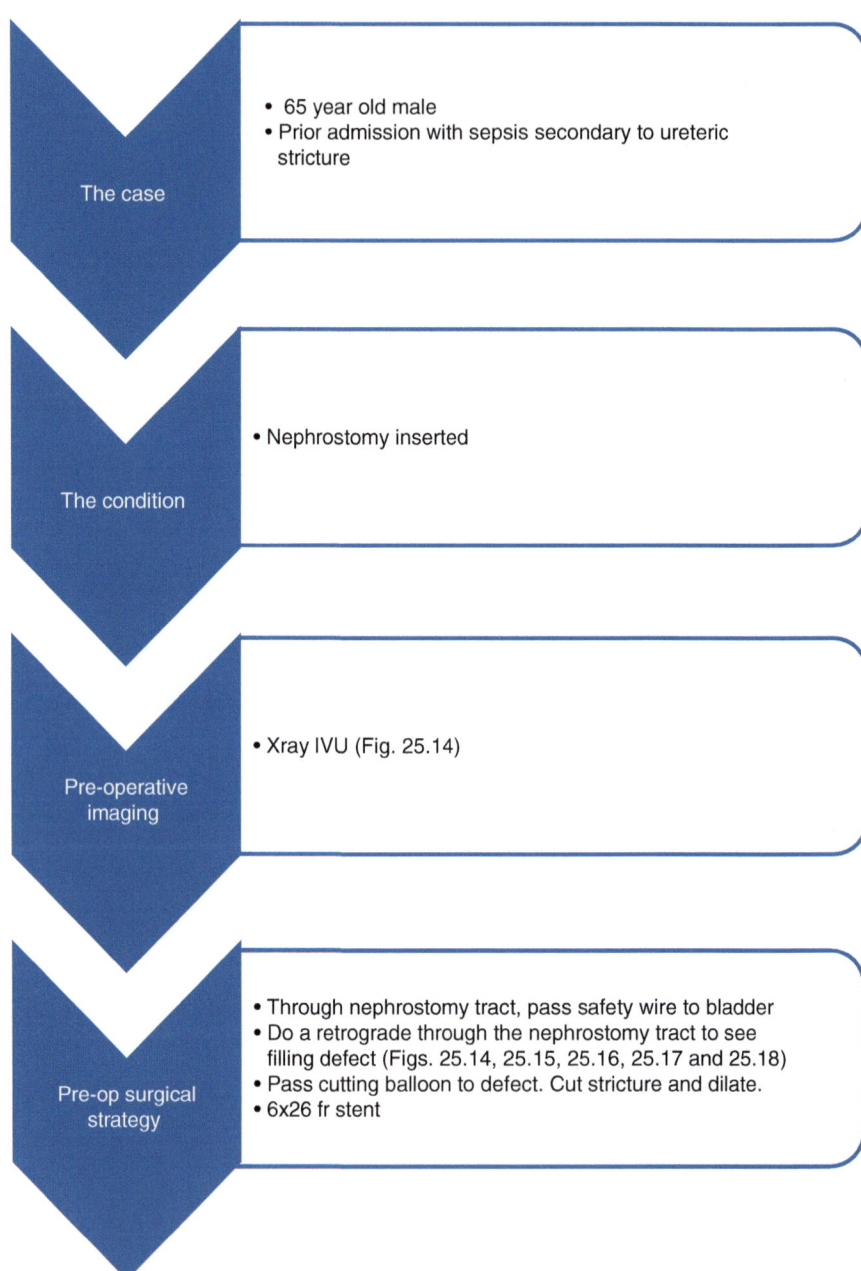

The case
- 65 year old male
- Prior admission with sepsis secondary to ureteric stricture

The condition
- Nephrostomy inserted

Pre-operative imaging
- Xray IVU (Fig. 25.14)

Pre-op surgical strategy
- Through nephrostomy tract, pass safety wire to bladder
- Do a retrograde through the nephrostomy tract to see filling defect (Figs. 25.14, 25.15, 25.16, 25.17 and 25.18)
- Pass cutting balloon to defect. Cut stricture and dilate.
- 6x26 fr stent

Factors which may limit success
Long strictures (> 1 cm)
Ischemic / radiation etiology
Impaired renal function
Mid-ureteral location
"Old" strictures (> 6 months)
Ureteroenteric strictures

Fig. 25.14 Pre operative IVU

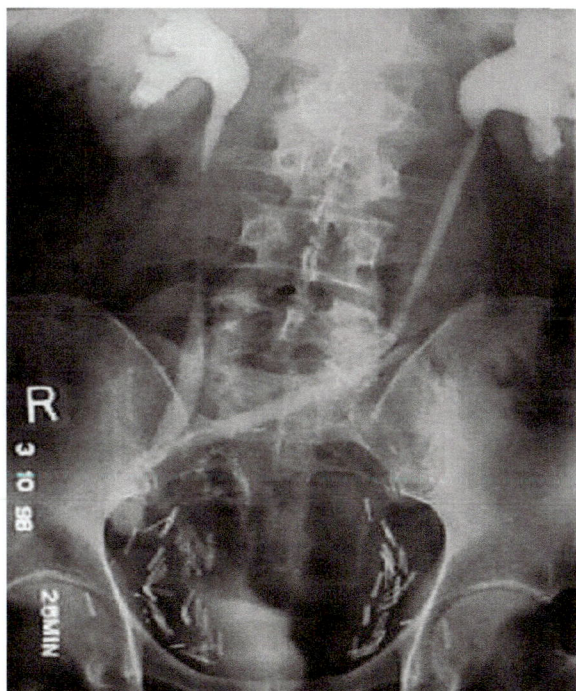

Fig. 25.15 Antegrade
ureterogram

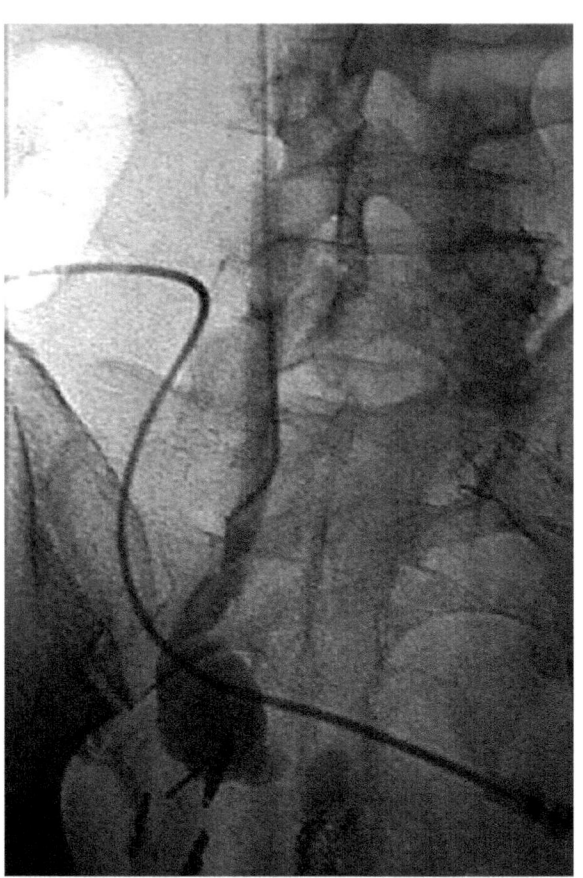

Fig. 25.16 Wire across ureteric stricture

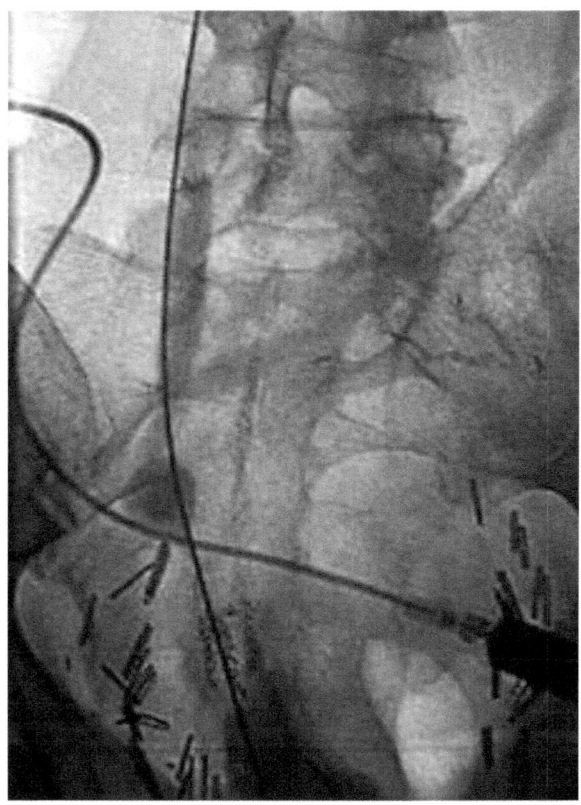

Fig. 25.17 Cutting balloon passed up retrogradely

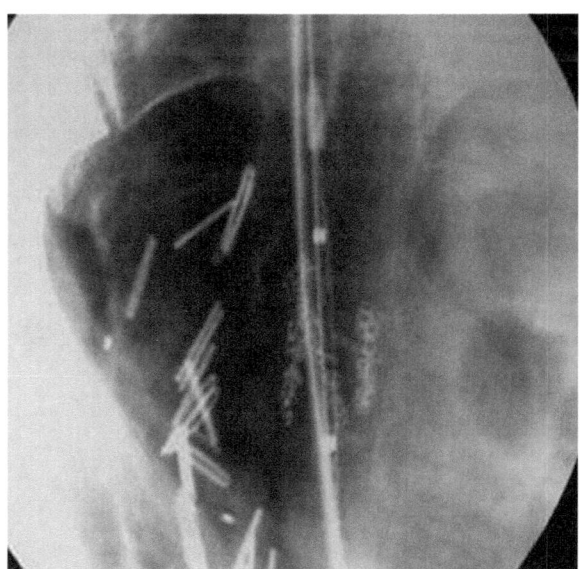

Fig. 25.18 Balloon
dilation

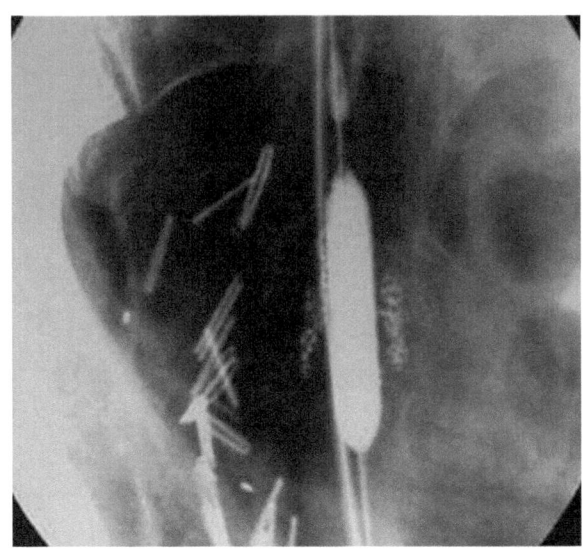

References

Banner MP, Pollack HM. Dilatation of ureteral stenoses: techniques and experience in 44 patients. AJR Am J Roentgenol. 1984;143(4):789–93.

Banner MP, Pollack HM, Ring EJ, Wein AJ. Catheter dilatation of benign ureteral strictures. Radiology. 1983;147(2):427–33.

Chang R, Marshall FF. Management of ureteroscopic injuries. J Urol. 1987;137(6):1132–5.

Finnerty DP, Trulock TS, Berkman W, Walton KN. Transluminal balloon dilation of ureteral strictures. J Urol. 1984;131(6):1056–60.

Glanz S, Gordon DH, Butt K, Rubin B, Hong J, Sclafani SJ. Percutaneous transrenal balloon dilatation of the ureter. Radiology. 1983;149(1):101–4.

O'Brien WM, Maxted WC, Pahira JJ. Ureteral stricture: experience with 31 cases. J Urol. 1988;140(4):737–40.

Wolf JS Jr, Elashry OM, Clayman RV. Long-term results of endoureterotomy for benign ureteral and ureteroenteric strictures. J Urol. 1997;158(3 Pt 1):759–64.

Surgical Strategy for Bladder Stones

26

26.1 Management Options for Bladder Stones

Bladder stones are rare and most cases occur in adult men with bladder outlet obstruction. Different rates of calculus-free patients are described in each of them, as follows: extracorporeal shock wave lithotripsy (75-100%), transurethral cystolithotripsy (63-100%), percutaneous cystolithotripsy (89-100%) and open surgery (100 %). (Torcelli, 2013).

The percutaneous approach has lower morbidity, with similar results to the transurethral treatment, while extracorporeal lithotripsy has the lowest rate of elimination of calculi and is reserved for patients at high surgical risk (Torcelli, 2013).

Both trans-urethral and percutaneous lithotripsy were efficacy for stone fragmentation although the last one was suggested to avoid urethral injuries. Holmiun:Yag laser lithotripsy has made stone fragmentation feasible by using local anesthesia however in selected patients only. (Cicone, 2018)

26.2   Case 1 Bladder Stones

The case
- 73 year old male, elevated BMI
- Haematuria and minimal LUTS.
- Past medical history – high BMI
- Prev Ca Prostate + DXT, now on androgen deprivation therapy

The condition
- Stone 4x3 cm on CT
- Prev Ca Prostate + DXT
- Androgen deprivation therapy
- Not properly emptying bladder

Pre-operative imaging
- CT KUB
- Old MRI
- Figures 26.1 and 26.2

Pre-op surgical strategy
- Check table can take weight
- Have extra long resectoscope in theatre with clutton sounds
- Dilate urethra
- Laser bladder stone first, start at 0.8/10 and increase, fragment, and extract
- Laser to prostate - HOLEP settings

The equipment

- HOLEP Laser
- Rigid cystoscope and ureteric catheter or HOLEP set with Bridge
- Long resectoscope/ Stone punch on standby and clutton sounds

The strategy

- EUA, stiff bladder neck
- Rigid cystoscope in, with bridge
- Dilate urethra wityh clutton sounds up to 26 fr
- Be wary of the median lobe, this can bleed the most, especially when using holep to laser
- Laser bladder stone first- using holep settings of 0.4J/ 20 Hz, dust stone and keep washing out bladder/ extracting the fragments using an Ellick
- HOLEP of prostate as 2nd procecdure

The outcome

- Stone fully cleared
- Chase stone type.
- Dietary advice including BAUS information leaflet.
- TFTs, Calcium, Urate.

Fig. 26.1 Bladder stone
on non-contrast CT

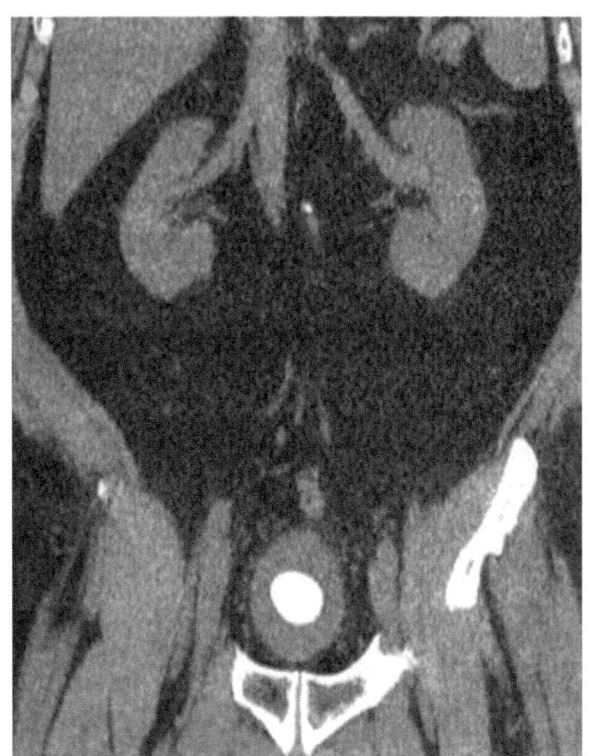

Fig. 26.2 MRI of the prostate

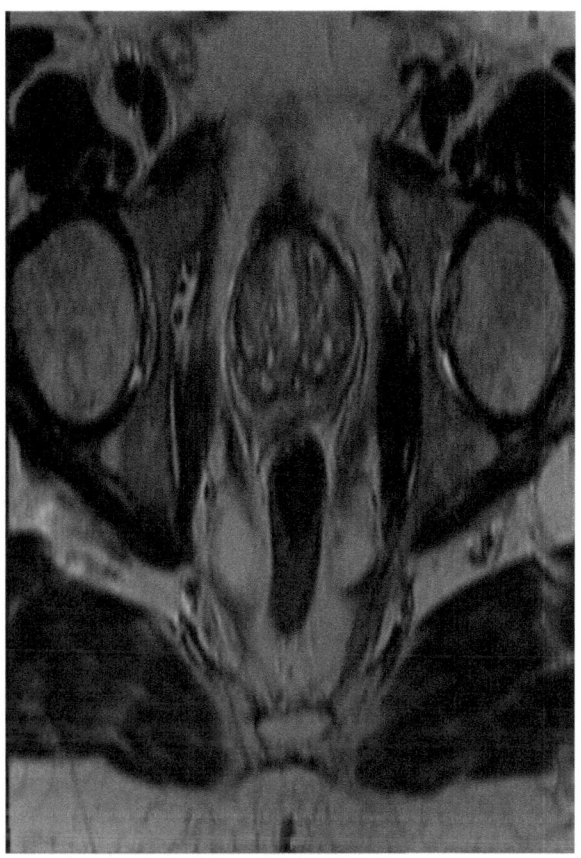

26.3   Laparoscopic Approach to Bladder Stones

Roslan determined the feasibility and safety of performing transvesical laparoendoscopic single-site surgery (T-LESS) in patients with medium-size, hard stones or multiple stones with high burden (Roslan, 2019). In this case series study, 12 patients (11 males and one female) with a mean age of 66.8 years were operated on from February 2016 to May 2017 due to bladder calculi, using the T-LESS approach with a single-port device (Tri-Port +, Olympus, Germany) (Roslan, 2019).

Indications for this procedure were hard, medium-size, solitary stones after previous unsuccessful endoscopic lithotripsy or the presence of multiple high-burden stones (Roslan, 2019). In two patients, additional procedures (diverticulectomy or a ureterocele incision) were performed simultaneously (Roslan, 2019).

All stones were removed intact. No serious complications were observed. The mean operative time was 46 min and the postoperative hospital stay was 22 h (Roslan, 2019). The mean diameter of the largest stone and the mean stone volume of each case were 24 mm and 11 cm3, respectively (Roslan, 2019). At the mean follow-up time of 15 months, there was significant improvement of the symptoms.

The T-LESS technique is an efficient, safe and minimally invasive procedure for intact bladder stone removal in selected patients (Roslan, 2019). The method avoids the risk of urethral injury. Nevertheless, further investigation is needed to assess the wider applicability of the procedure (Roslan, 2019).

References

Torricelli FCM, Mazzucchi E, Danilovic A, Coelho RF, Srougi M. Surgical management of bladder stones: literature review. Rev Col Bras Cir. 2013;40(3):227–33.

Cicione A, DE Nunzio C, Posti SMRDA, Lima E, Tubaro A, Balloni F. Bladder stone management: an update. Minerva Urol Nefrol. 2018;70(1):53–65.

Roslan M, Przudzik M, Borowik M. Endoscopic intact removal of medium-size- or multiple bladder stones with the use of transvesical laparoendoscopic single-site surgery. World J Urol. 2019;37(2):373–8.

Surgical Strategy for a Bulbourethral Stricture

27.1 Causes of Urethral Stricture

Urethral strictures

The traumatic injury of patients accounted for 52.4% (96/183), in which the pelvic fracture accounted for 35.5% (65/183) and the straddle injury accounted for 16.9% (31/183).

There were 54 cases of iatrogenic injury (29.5%). The posterior urethral stricture accounted for 45.9% (84/183), followed by the anterior urethral stricture (44.8%, 82/183) and the stenosis (6.6%, 12/183). (Chen, 2018).

A total of 99 patients (54.1%) received the end to end anastomosis, and 40 (21.9%) were treated with intracavitary surgery, such as endoscopic holmium laser, cold knife incision, endoscopic electroknife scar removal, balloon dilation, and urethral dilation.

In the patients over 65-years old, the urethral stricture rate was 14.8% and the complication rate (70.4%) for transurethral resection of the prostate (TURP) was significantly higher than that of all samples (P<0.01).

(Chen, 2018)

S. S. Goonewardene et al., *Surgical Strategies in Endourology for Stone Disease*, https://doi.org/10.1007/978-3-030-82143-2_27

27.2   Case 1

The case
- Flexi-bulbar urethral stricture
- IPSS score is 23 with a quality of life score of 5
- Storage LUTS
- PSA 1.82

The condition
- 70 year old male
- Recurrent bulbourethral stricture
- Symptoms of frequency, urgency and incomplete emptying

Pre-operative imaging
- CT KUB (Figs. 27.1 and 27.2)

The equipment

- HOLEP set and bridge
- CLutton sounds and long resectoscope, Bipolar resectoscope on standby

The strategy

- EUA (Figs. 27.3, 27.4, 27.5 and 27.6)
- Rigid cystoscope in, with bridge
- Assess prostate, urethra and bladder.
- If the Verumontanum is long, with a high bladder neck, the HOLEP will be difficult.
- Resectoscope in, 100 W, 2J energy settings
- Identify UOs and stay clear. Assess prostate, to see if trilobar or bilobar
- Resect median lobe, then lateral lobes.
- Morcellate, then assess the bladder to ensure no perforation
- 3 way catheter with irrigation.
- TWOC in 24 hours

The difficulties

- UOs can be adjacent to the median lobe or on the median love- assess carefully and laser around.
- There may not be enough of a median lobe to create a channel.
- Vascular prostates- take your time and diathermise as you go.
- It is very easy to loose orientation within the prostate - always define and keep to your plane- you do not want to go back and re-laser to create the plane/ remove residual prostate tissue.
- Dual treatment, both bipolar resection and HOLEP- the mushroom hybrid methodlaser enough to keep lobes tethered. If a large prostate, you may not be able to reach the lobes to morcellate. Resect with the bipolar resectoscope if that is an issue.
- The other difficulty is reaching lobes- use the long resectoscope if needs be
- If in a difficult position, do not do lobectomy- it will not work.

The outcome

- Prostate successfully resected
- Histology benign
- Patient attended 3 months later for flows and PVR- good flow rate and no PVR.

Fig. 27.1 CT
demonstrating upper tracts
negative

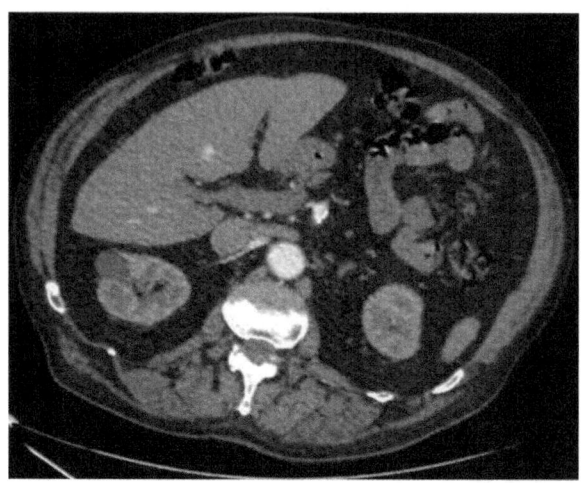

Fig. 27.2 Large volume
bladder on CT

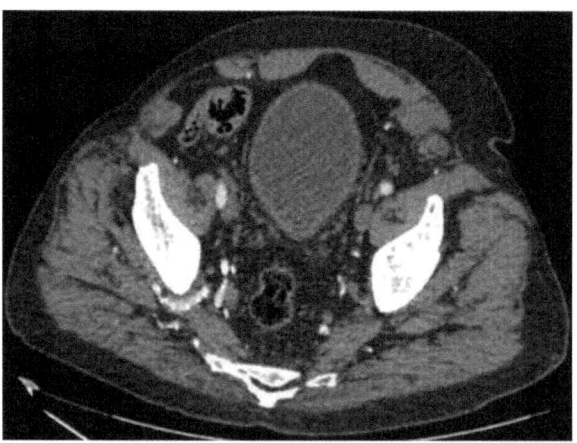

Fig. 27.3 A Bulbourethral Stricture

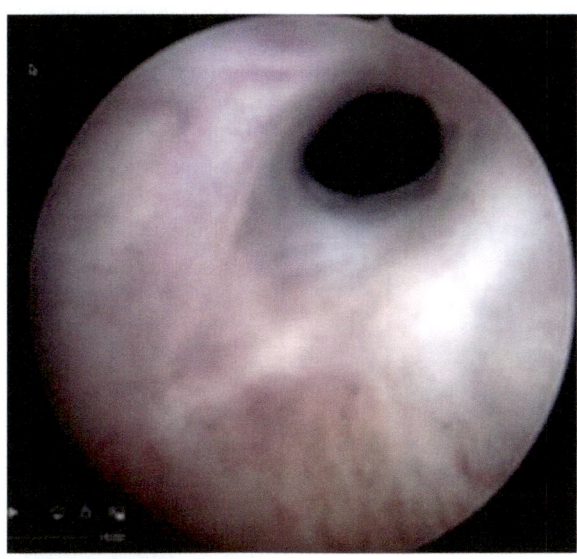

Fig. 27.4 Pass a wire across the stricture

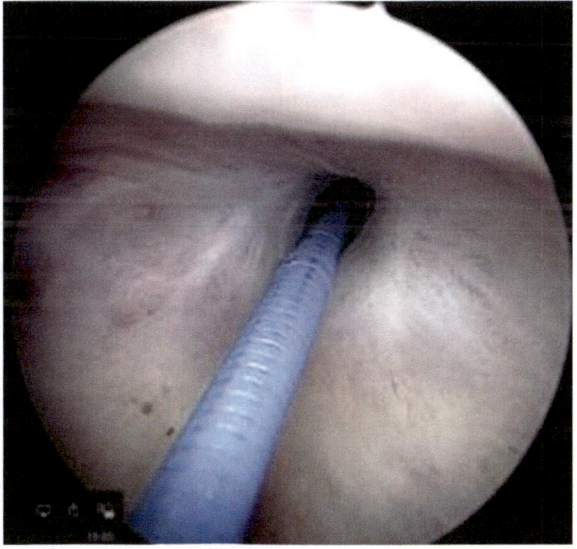

Fig. 27.5 Open up the stricture with a serrated blade

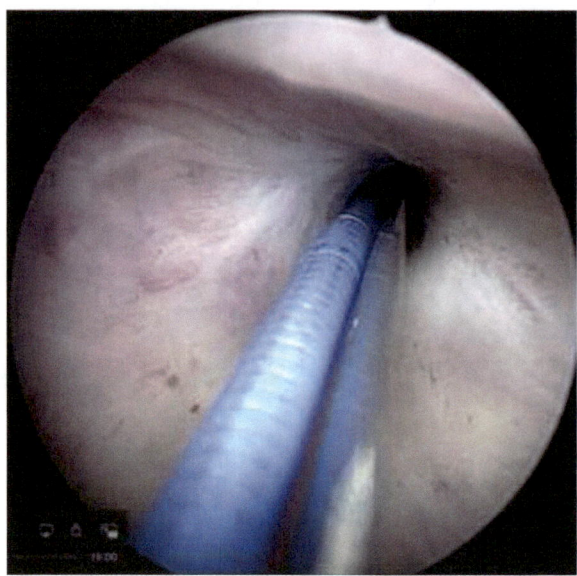

Fig. 27.6 Opening up the stricture

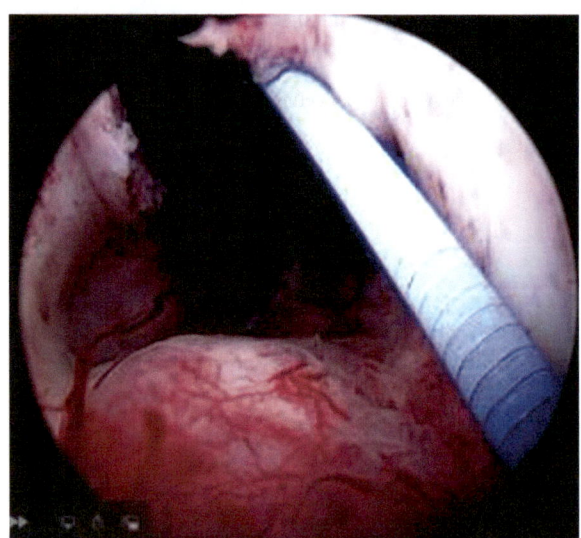

Reference

Chen C, Zeng M, Xue R, Wang G, Gao Z, Yuan W, Tang Z. Causes and management for male urethral stricture. Zhong Nan Da Xue Xue Bao Yi Xue Ban. 2018;43(5):520–7.

Index

© The Editor(s) (if applicable) and The Author(s), under exclusive license to
Springer Nature Switzerland AG 2021
S. S. Goonewardene et al., *Surgical Strategies in Endourology for Stone Disease*,
https://doi.org/10.1007/978-3-030-82143-2

GPSR Compliance

The European Union's (EU) General Product Safety Regulation (GPSR) is a set of rules that requires consumer products to be safe and our obligations to ensure this.

If you have any concerns about our products, you can contact us on ProductSafety@springernature.com

In case Publisher is established outside the EU, the EU authorized representative is:

Springer Nature Customer Service Center GmbH
Europaplatz 3
69115 Heidelberg, Germany

Batch number: 10091867

Printed by Printforce, the Netherlands